Bipolar Hell

*How I Lost My Mind and
Became a Secret Agent*

Andrew McLean

Dedication

As you'll discover when you read the pages that follow, there are many people that are intertwined in the crazy story that I am about to tell. And there have been many people that have supported me on my path to recovery, both friends and family.

However, there's one character who almost plays as big a part as me - Yuni, my girlfriend during my manic episode in Bali in 2019.

Yuni, this book is dedicated to you.

Table of Contents

Prologue

I bolted towards the nearest door, leaving my flip-flops behind as I dashed toward the beach. The beach was safe, a place I could hide in plain sight.

I approached a small beachside bar and hid there for a while, concealing myself among the tourists and locals.

I have to talk to Yuni, my girlfriend.

Quickly, I shuffled through my pockets to reveal a piece of paper with the most important phone numbers that I had written down the day before. However, another problem awaited me: my phone battery was dead.

My breath caught, I wondered what I should do now.

I had to tell Yuni that our safe house, the villa in Berawa, was no longer safe and that she shouldn't return there. Despite my desperation, no one on the beach agreed to lend me their phone to make a call - I was dumbfounded.

My mind was racing. I could only trust Balinese people, so when a man appeared out of nowhere and said that he was from Sumbawa, I freaked out and ran for it.

The world was caving in on my reality.

What was real, what was fake? I didn't know how to distinguish between either of them.

There was nothing that I could be sure of, nor was there anywhere that I felt safe.

Maybe I could stay on the beach - maybe Yuni would find me. I mean, who would attack someone on the beach in broad daylight? But I wasn't going to take any chances.

I pondered whether I should run south towards Kuta or north towards Canggu. Going north would mean going past Finns, the beach club where I had been with Yuni and my friend Ketut the day before, and possibly being recognized!

My mind was a tumbling mess, but I somehow felt that all my actions were my own, and every move that I made needed to be calculated. I felt my life depended on my next decision.

I was in the middle of the single craziest day of my life.

Chapter 1: Bali, The Island of My Dreams

"Fuck, Andy" Jacqui muttered under her breath. She gave me a second glance as she continued, "You should've done something about this months ago!".

She was talking about the fact I'd been diagnosed with bipolar disorder, but I'd never mentioned it to her until that point on a random Thursday afternoon in September 2018.

Yeah, sure. I could feel myself grimacing at the thought as I took a deep breath and stared out the window of Jacqui's apartment in downtown Malmo, Sweden. I was with my best friend from university in New Zealand, where I grew up, and my family still lived.

I'd been in London for the summer, and it had been long and lonely. Being with my friend, someone who knew me so well, was such a good feeling.

There are always certain things that we believe we should have done long ago. For example, that new diet or workout regime! We might tell ourselves that we regret not sitting under the sun for longer or fixing our sleep cycles, but here's the catch.

If we all did what we were supposed to be doing, our lives wouldn't be as unpredictable as they turned out to be. Life makes so much more sense when looking in the rear-view mirror.

And while a perfect life path sounds rather ideal, in my case, many minor crashes ultimately led me to where I still am today – in Bali, Indonesia.

The year before, in November 2017, I had been admitted to The Priory, an expensive private psychiatric hospital in London. I went there voluntarily after some work colleagues became concerned about my state of mind.

My stay lasted almost a month, ultimately costing me my job and, more importantly, the social fabric of my being. I also didn't understand what being bipolar meant other than that I had to swallow a cocktail of pills each day.

I spent the next nine months looking for work in an attempt to be normal again, but it proved to be a fruitless search. With loneliness mustering itself in the pits of my heart and unemployment bringing my morale down, it was that meeting with Jacqui that convinced me to move to Bali, a place where I had spent countless memorable days over the preceding five years.

Now, you may ask why I chose Bali in particular.

I can respond with a quote.

> "Old God sure was in a good mood when he made this place."
> **— Hunter S. Thompson, The Rum Diary**

Back in 2013, in London, my company granted me a six-month sabbatical, and after a few weeks back home in New Zealand, I landed in Bali with no real plan. I had a mate that lived there, and his place was like a sanctuary for me. I chilled, read books, and swam each day.

And boy, did I need it!

In the year since my wife committed suicide, I'd become a train wreck.

I was performing on the outside and delivered two big projects at work, but I was beyond broken on the inside. I was battling the alcoholism that comes with grief and loneliness.

Yet Bali proved to be the perfect place to recover. Two of the three months I spent in Indonesia before returning to London were in Bali, known as the Island of the Gods.

By the end of my time there, I was able to experience such intense spiritual healing that I felt fully recovered from all my depression and alcoholism. So I left Bali with great memories and was excited about what lay ahead.

Over the next few years, I frequently retreated to Bali whenever I wanted to take a whiff away from the tyranny of life. Over my many trips, I came to make a terrific group of Balinese friends.

And so you might think, why not go home to New Zealand in a moment of crisis? Bali was the most obvious choice for me. It was cheap, I had friends to stay with, and it had served me well more than once.

★ ★ ★

Two days of deep conversation with Jacqui in Malmo made me realize I hadn't invested any time in understanding what bipolar disorder was. The psychiatrist at The Priory hadn't explained it to me in any way other than suggesting a book I could read about overcoming mood swings.

So, upon arriving in Bali, I sought a local psychiatrist to help me understand it all. Within a few days, I made an appointment with Dr. Monika Joy Reverger, reputed to be the leading psychiatrist on the island.

"Socialization is a big aspect playing in your mental state," Dr. Joy said.

I agreed. I had been alone each weekday during the summer in London while everyone else was at work, disconnected from my social circle.

As I explained to Dr. Joy how my life in London had been since I lost my job, she suggested that loneliness affected my social battery and emotional state. Having this insight into myself through the eyes of someone professionally capable came as an immense relief.

That a lack of socialization was affecting me day-to-day explained everything. Dr. Joy confirmed she would keep me on the same medication dosages that I'd been given at The Priory and said she'd monitor it each month.

★ ★ ★

I always thought I had a pretty normal life before admitting to The Priory. I had no inkling that I might have a mental illness, even though I had a nasty bout of depression in my early twenties. However, that's what we keep thinking about ourselves, don't we?

It's never too bad until it gets bad.

I had lived in London since 2005 and forged a successful career working for Investec, a bank that originated in South Africa. Through all the grind and hard work, I acquired three apartments and, most importantly, a sense of financial security. I played sports, had a great group of friends, ran the London marathon, and completed my MBA.

You know, the things ordinary people do.

I also found love. In 2010, I tied the knot with a girl named Rima. My life was complete with a lovely apartment in Central London and a loving partner. As if there was nothing more I'd want to cherish for the rest of my life.

But, odd how things take horrible turns, huh?

In 2012, Rima took her own life, a tragedy that sent me to the deepest pits of depression over the year that followed. By mid-2013, I was struggling to cope with life and developed a strong attachment to alcohol.

I was making poor decisions, the worst being moving out of my apartment in an area I loved just because a friend said it was a good idea. As I moved into a new area, Kilburn, that I hated, every kiss of wine tasted like my last chance at a better life.

Yet somehow, I realized it was not the solution, and much to my relief, my boss instinctively also knew that I needed a break from London life. The six-month sabbatical that Jamie gave me in 2013 was oh-so-needed.

★ ★ ★

Jamie was the best boss I have ever had. We were the best of mates.

When I was admitted to The Priory in 2017, his concern for my well-being was the deciding factor in my decision to go there. He suspected I might be suffering from PTSD, and while his diagnosis was wrong, his intuition was spot on.

The Priory caught everyone by surprise, me included. Only Jamie and my then-boss Chris saw the signs that I was getting out of control, both at work and in the text messages that I was sending.

But, in my mind, work and life had been going well; it's amazing what others that care about you can see that you can't. This feeling led me to buy a new car and move out of London for a better lifestyle.

It was almost like I had lost my attachment to any intangible aspect of my life.

Little did I know that a long-pending mania had crept into my life, slowly yet surely. My parents found out about me being in The Priory only after I 'escaped' from there. Until then, only Jamie, Chris, and Nick, my best friend in London, knew what was happening.

It must have come as a major shock to my family back in New Zealand, yet only Mum sought to find out what was going on, and Jamie did his best to explain what had happened. And the only person from work that came to visit me was James, another great mate from Investec.

Immediately after my month at The Priory, I went home to New Zealand for Christmas, and as best as I can remember, my family had little to say to me. I guess they were just happy to see me, and, in reality, none of us knew that I was bipolar because, at that point, the psychiatrist at The Priory had only said my mind was in a 'mixed state'.

It took the severe manic episode I had in Bali in 2019, which is the real reason for writing this book, for my family to get involved with my illness. It was an SOS call from my girlfriend to say she couldn't cope with me on her own, and my being in the psychiatric ward of a public hospital in a foreign land that made them wake up to the fact there was a serious problem.

★ ★ ★

December 2018 - Ubud, Bali

From that decision in Malmo to leave London, it was all done in a couple of days. I sold my car, left my apartment in Kilburn for my friend Terry to live in, and boarded a plane from Heathrow.

The only Balinese friend I told about my plan was Yani, someone I had stayed with earlier in the year. She had a rental apartment across the rice fields from her house in Ubud, meaning I had the perfect place to land.

Ubud is a town an hour inland from Bali's famous beaches, and its name literally translates as medicine.

It has a vibrant yoga community and is dominated by health-food cafes rather than lively bars.

The first two months in Ubud were about getting healthy and refraining from alcohol. Each day Yani and I would have a morning walk together and then go to a meditation class at Radiantly Alive.

Best of all, there were always people at her house that I could chat and eat with. Yani's house was almost like a socialization hub that was on tap, a bit like a beer!

And because I had other friends in Ubud, like Wayan and Kadek, I soon realized that Bali might be where I wanted to grow old. However, as Dad reminded me when he visited in November, I had to get a job to keep my mind ticking over if I wanted to stay in Bali.

It's funny how things happen. One day, a few weeks after Dad said that, I was chatting to an English guy called Justin, and after asking him what work he might do in Bali if he stayed, he said to me, "well, you'd obviously teach English".

A couple of days later, I was in a taxi when I thought of Justin's comment. I went online and found a company in Denpasar called 'English First,' a global educational company that specializes in language training. It turned out that it was actively hiring.

While working in Denpasar, Bali's biggest city and a 45-minute motorcycle ride from Ubud didn't particularly thrill me, I figured my chances of getting hired were decent. After that, it was a surprisingly easy process. Dad's 'get-a-job' box was ticked.

After the horrible nine months I had endured living in London after The Priory and feeling totally worthless, I finally felt like something good was going on in my life - something worth living for. And, as I have often found in life, good fortune happens simultaneously in more ways than one.

★ ★ ★

On the same day that I had my interview with English First, I went on a second date with an Indonesian girl called Yuni, not to be confused with Yani, and soon we were meeting once a week.

Meeting Yuni helped me reconnect with my life again, helping me with the socialization I needed oh-so-desperately. I had found what had been missing! We ended up taking a romantic trip together to a nearby island a couple of weeks later, and by New Year's Eve, I had found love again, even if I didn't express it to her at the time.

Yuni was a solo mother from Java, the island to the west of Bali, and she lived with her mum and son. Immediately, I knew she was knowledgeable and bright, albeit a few years younger than me. She held down an excellent job, providing her with the financial independence to do as she pleased.

She was short, petite, and had a jaw-dropping smile. Our mutual love for traveling and watching sunsets drew me to her. After my job at English First was confirmed, I decided that I needed to move closer to my office, so I asked Yuni, "How about I live near you?".

She was delighted to hear this, and I found a lovely apartment ten minutes from her house in Kerobokan. So as I started my new job, we began seeing each other on most days for dinner.

It had been almost seven years since Rima passed away, and Yuni was my first relationship after that. It's not as if I hadn't met other women, but I'd found the whole dating process to be beyond difficult, especially in London.

I can make a million excuses for not meeting anyone, but perhaps it just wasn't meant to be. Life sometimes is more about being in the right place at the right time.

It felt amazing to be with Yuni, and I knew I wanted her in my life - I had fallen head over heels for her. She gave me hope as to why life had another chance at being great again, and I wanted her to be there with me the entire time.

The previous seven years had undoubtedly been forlorn, having no companion to lean on in my tough times. Love had been severely lacking in my life, and

I only came to that again after finding Yuni, who reignited my belief in second love.

She made me feel safe in her arms, and I knew nothing could get to me if I had her support and companionship throughout this journey.

It's hard for me to describe how transformative this time was, yet I'm trying to scribble as much of my unkempt mind onto this page as possible. Man tries, fails, and then gets back up to try again – which I believed to be only fictional or magical. After all that I had been through, I was on the road to giving up on life, but in 2018 and 2019, Bali proved that second chances exist.

There are *always* second chances.

Chapter 2: Coming Clean About My Illness

February 2019

My only Balinese friend that knew about my bipolar was Yani, not that she really knew what it meant. I'd not mentioned it to Yuni, fearing she would reject me.

It was a dinner in Ubud just before starting my new job that I realized I had to come clean with Yuni. That dinner was with Jacqui, who was holidaying in Ubud, and I'd arranged for Yuni and I to dine with her and her friend.

An hour before we met Jacqui, I told Yuni about my mental health condition. I figured that after three months together, it was safe to do so. It turned out that this revelation didn't surprise her as she had read my blog post about it. Who doesn't Google their new boyfriend?

"I love you and care about you, Andy." Yuni's eyes teared up as we spoke about my illness. She continued, stroking my cheek lovingly, "I'll be on this journey with you. You are not alone. Let's live life together".

My relief was palpable. Job done!

★ ★ ★

With Yuni on my side, it was time to get to work, and immediately I reveled in my new job teaching English. I got on famously with the Balinese office staff, and soon my student ratings were off the charts. Remember by this point I hadn't done a day's work for more than a year, so it was a feeling of going from worthless to valuable almost overnight.

Within a few days in my new workplace, I realized that I was not only doing something I was good at, but it was also something that I absolutely loved!

It was all new to me, and I felt energized. I was teaching in a virtual classroom with students from around the globe - from China, South America, Europe, and other countries that I would never have had contact with while working for a bank in London.

I had spent fifteen years working in the corporate sector on projects inside the bank, so I barely knew commerce outside of my limited working life. Yet, somehow, these new daily conversations with my students gave me an insight into what the rest of the world was up to.

They were exciting times.

I also realized that I was not only teaching these students how to read and converse in English, but also teaching them about other valuable life skills because I had so much of my experience to draw on. Through my lessons, my students could learn how to navigate job interviews and write resumes, which would help them later in their lives.

And I was so glad to be a part of their journeys - it felt relevant and meaningful. To act as a source of guidance to all these students who looked up to me through the glance of inspiration, as I had often done with younger colleagues back at the bank in London, was something truly special.

One attraction of accepting the teaching job at English First was that it came with a work permit, which is a rarity in Bali. I figured it was a formality but, as I will mention later, this was far from the case.

★ ★ ★

Over Easter of 2019, Yuni and I took a trip to the Gili Islands in Lombok, the next-door province east of Bali. It turned out to be a magical few days together.

Although she had previously worked for many years at a beach resort in Sulawesi, another part of Indonesia, Yuni was not a confident swimmer. So we spent many hours on Gili Meno working on this and having many laughs along the way.

I was so enthralled by the beauty of Gili Meno, the least-visited of the three islands in the Gili group, that I struck up a conversation with Yuni about possibly starting a new venture there.

"I think we could open a coffee shop here." I looked at Yuni with loving eyes as she laughed at my suggestion, not mockingly, but gleefully.

"What about opening a new English training course center?"

"Or a water sports business?"

The opportunities seemed endless as they rolled off my tongue. My life, our life, was just about to begin, or at least I thought so.

★ ★ ★

May 2019 - The start of a monumental mental meltdown

When I had started with English First back in February, they'd booked a flight to Singapore for me to collect my work permit, and the day before I was due to fly, they said it wasn't ready. "No worries," I said, knowing that these things don't always go to plan.

However, it was now May, and the issue was still unsolved. It had been bothering me for several weeks now. Simply put, I had a contract with a reputable employer with dozens of other foreign staff, yet somehow my visa was lost somewhere in the ether.

I'd had several meetings with Ria from HR and Kumara, my boss, yet no progress was being made. I'd successfully applied for several visas to different countries in the past so, instinctively, I knew something was wrong.

Worried and perplexed, I sought guidance from Yuni, who had years of experience working in HR in Indonesia. She had a profound knowledge of the work permit process for foreigners. As she slowly asked me questions and asked to see my documentation, her ears perked up, and her eyes narrowed. It was a look I dreaded seeing.

Much to my dismay, Yuni also believed something was unusually wrong with my visa situation. Of course, this shouldn't have been a big deal, but that's not how it felt.

Concerned, I had become extremely suspicious of the agent handling my application, a lady called Ayu, who was based in Surabaya, a Javanese city where our head office was located. Too many so-called 'reasons' for the delay in processing my work permit simply didn't make sense, and I took my feelings out on Kumara, who was not just my boss but also a great friend.

Kumara took the full force of my anger as I demanded that she find a better agent to process my work permit.

I am so grateful that she withstood my tirade, and somehow, remarkably, we are still good friends today.

At the same time, I had been doing a lot of overtime and had little to no time left for myself. Whatever leisure time I had, I would spend it trying to fix the issue with my visa – which wasn't bearing any fruit either. Stress and fatigue kept nibbling on the tendons in my mind, which sent my emotional state spiraling out of control with its intensity.

If you stretch an elastic band more than its capability, it is bound to break. If I try to explain this analogy to others, they remind me I'm not a material object like an elastic band. That's the thing, isn't it? Even if something simple as a band can break, why can't a complex bundle of blood and nerves, aka humans, break too?

The stress manifested itself in several ways. I had lost interest in exercising and felt increasingly fatigued and cramped. Other than that, I wasn't eating well, which is never a good sign for anyone in distress. Although I didn't realize it then, I was losing quite a lot of weight. You could see the apprehension in my eyes and my entire demeanor!

★ ★ ★

When I first met Dr. Joy, she had prescribed me an antidepressant, an antipsychotic, and a mood stabilizer, and she had progressively begun reducing my medication after each monthly meeting. Because of how closely she monitored me, by January 2019, I thought I could quit it altogether.

"We're going to be reducing your medication to just a small dosage of an antidepressant. Maybe that's a good step for you, Andy."

"Are you sure, Dr. Joy?" I asked.

She reasoned, fixing her posture confidently, "If we can avoid a depressive episode, it will be unlikely that you experience a manic one like you had at The Priory."

By this juncture and after coming to feel that a doctor finally had taken the time to talk to me and understand me, I trusted Dr. Joy implicitly and I'm pretty sure that she also trusted me.

I had told Dr. Joy about Yuni and how I was starting my job at English First. With this news and seeing a big smile on my face, she must have been so confident, and happy, that I was on a good path.

★ ★ ★

Over the second weekend in May, I went to New Zealand for the auspicious Mother's Day, which was on the same date as Mum's birthday. It was a great time spent with my family, and I seemed to connect well with them throughout my time there.

Everyone threw remarks about how well I was doing.

"Andrew, you seem like you've been doing great!" Mum said.

"Andy seems to be recovering so well!" one friend said.

It sure felt like I was doing well, and it was, in my mind, the perfect weekend. Mum especially had been so happy to see me, as it had been a surprise visit.

Upon returning to Bali, I barely slept properly over those next few days. From the airport, on Monday, I went back to meet Yuni at my apartment, and, as she later told me, I was babbling on about something she knew nothing about.

A peaceful slumber was missing from my routine, and over the next week, I couldn't manage it. And all I could think about was that damned work permit. Little did I know how it was affecting my mental state.

I went into that next week as normal, scoring high marks in my teaching, but when I had to go to work on Saturday morning, I realized I was in no state to teach, having barely slept the whole week. The world around me kept spinning, sending me into a spiral of emotions as I wondered how I had ended up feeling like this.

While many things had changed for the better since my time in The Priory, I soon discovered that too much change, whether good or bad, can be overwhelming. We often undermine the importance of overwhelming situations - which have the potential to dazzle us in quite unpreferable ways.

My new life was fast-paced, and I could do nothing to fix the pace. Undoubtedly, this new life in Bali was exciting and mind-blowing in the best possible way, yet it proved to be something that could deter me and my energy levels.

I felt like I needed something to calm myself down. I told Christian, the manager, that I didn't feel well and needed to go home. And despite feeling frazzled in a way that I had never felt before, I somehow managed to drive my motorbike the twenty minutes back to my apartment.

I was in terrible shape, so I called Dr. Joy, disturbing her at home on a Saturday morning. "Joy, I need something to sedate me."

She said, "Okay, collect it from Siloam", a hospital in Kuta around twenty minutes from where I lived in Kerobokan. I was in no shape to drive, so I took a taxi.

I took another taxi to return to my apartment and called Yuni to tell her what had happened. I barely remember the rest of that day, Saturday, May 18, 2019.

Sunday was my day off and, feeling the way I was, I contacted work to say that I couldn't work on Monday. I knew I just had to survive the weekend until I could see Dr. Joy.

Chapter 3:
Entering Psychosis

I don't remember much about the weekend. I knew that I just had to sleep, and maybe I did. The only person who knows is Yuni and, most likely, she put me to bed on Sunday night before going home.

Seeing Dr Joy that Monday morning was a relief; I think I talked for half an hour non-stop. I told her how I was feeling and thinking, what was going on at work with my work-permit situation, and she prescribed me some new medication - remembering that I was barely on anything, whereas I was on a lot six months before.

She wrote a letter to English First explaining that I was in an unhealthy condition and needed to take a week off work. She also put strict guidelines around my working hours. I hugged her, and I was on my way.

★ ★ ★

Before my appointment with Dr. Joy that Monday morning, I had run a test on my laptop to see if the Wi-Fi at my apartment was strong enough to cope with the technical requirements of teaching English from home. I'd left it running while I was away, and after returning, I noticed a strange error message on the screen, which freaked the living lights out of me.

It was probably just a routine error message, but, by now, my mind was far from a normal state. You see, over the previous weeks, I had gotten myself deeply involved in my work-permit process, and I had come across certain documents that seemed fraudulent.

By that, I mean the documents for my application didn't seem authentic. After that, I not only became suspicious of Ayu, the agent handling my work-permit application, but also of Kumara.

When I saw that message on my laptop, I somehow concluded that the company was seeking to steal my identity. Though, my mind hadn't had enough time to react to the medication Dr. Joy had just prescribed me.

Instead, I felt that shit was about to go down. In the back of my mind, many scenarios ran through my conscience. What if the company was plotting against me?

Paranoia was harbored deep within my soul, and it ached to act on its own impulse.

I honestly believed that my company was out to get me.

Turning from my computer screen, I stared dumbfoundedly around my apartment, my happy home of the previous three months.

I have to clear out my bedroom.

They're out to get me.

One thought was all that I needed to spring right into action. I needed to ensure that there was nothing of concern in my room or any documents or important items. There had to be nothing in the room that could link straight to me and who I was.

As I locked the door and headed onto the street, I called Yuni and said nothing but, "Don't go into my apartment tonight. It's not safe."

Confused, she protested, "Whatever are you talking about, Andy?"

"Just... please." I sighed, my voice clearly expressing my concern, as I continued, "Just don't go there. I know you want answers, and so do I. I will tell you everything later. Just trust me."

And trust me, she did.

I felt terrible about not being able to discuss it more with Yuni, but there were other things of greater importance then which, I reasoned to myself, would directly harm both of us if I didn't think fast and act quickly.

★ ★ ★

Hailing a taxi, I went straight to Denpasar to buy
a new iPhone.

In my mind at that moment, my company could have
already infiltrated my identity, through my email
accounts and through my phone - and I couldn't have
them gaining permanent access to it.

My logic was that they'd successfully gained access
to my life by asking me to test their software and the
Wi-Fi connection at my apartment. I also realized that
the fingerprint scanner on the door at work could also
be a serious concern.

What could they possibly need that for?

What could they use my fingerprint for?

*Could they maybe steal my identity and fraudulently create
documents under my name through that fingerprint scanner
that is the fundamental connection someone would need?!*

Minute after minute, I could feel myself losing my
mind. I fell victim to my thinking and did everything
I could to reverse the situation and all the damage that
may have already been done.

Doing this meant I needed to buy a new phone, reset
all my passwords, and remove the touch ID sensor
from my phone and laptop. After doing so and paying
for the latest iPhone at Ibox in Denpasar, I walked

to Ibis Styles hotel and checked into a room. There was no way I could go back to my apartment that had possibly been infiltrated by whoever was trying to frame me!

I put all my important documents in the safe, including my old phone, which I knew had incriminating evidence against my company. I then walked next door to my other doctor's clinic and asked him to keep my passport safe with him.

I had to be sure.

I had to be safe.

Even though my life was flipping upside down, I still had to attend to my due obligations as a teacher. I had an English class to teach at UOB Bank that night as part of job with English First, and the thought of the staff there also conspiring against me in some kind of a fucked-up plan kept running through my head. However, I knew I had to act as normally as possible to fly under the radar.

Even though I arrived late, my first class went well. Nothing out of the ordinary happened until the second class of the day.

"Let's learn about–"

I stopped dead in my tracks as I stared at the two men in my class, texting more than they normally would. Fear began to foster within me as I thought, "Are they also part of this plan to conspire against me? Are they talking about it now as they sit in this class with me? What if English First put them purposefully in my class to watch me?"

I had to stop my mind from running loose.

However, the other part of my brain kept pushing odd and fearful thoughts into my head.

Who were they texting?

What were they reporting, and to whom do they report?

I sighed in distress. Shaking my head to reorient myself, I quickly jumped back into my teaching persona and did what I could to distract myself.

After class, it was always normal for students to openly discuss their lives - specifically, mine. It was OKAY to ask questions like, "Where are you headed after class, Mr. McLean?" or, "What is your girlfriend like, and where does she work?" - however, the suspicion in my head did not help my situation. I feared everyone and every question they had to ask about me.

Amid this mental turmoil, I did something out of the ordinary.

I went to see Yuni's sister and brother-in-law. They were surprised that I had taken the time to be there since I had only met them a handful of times before that visit. However, I stood on their doorstep because I believed I was in danger. That there was someone out there, planning to steal my identity.

As expected, Yuni was informed of my whereabouts and the condition I was in. She came to pick me up, no doubt bewildered by what was unfolding.

I needed Yuni to stay with me during this time, and she had left her mum and son at home by themselves to attend to me. She had never left them alone for the night, which made me realize how dire the situation had become.

Returning to my apartment was not an option, so we rented a hotel room in Umalas. It was imperative to be somewhere that we could be safe and that no one could find us. Yuni reasoned that it would help me to feel better.

Little did she know that there was no *getting better* for me. At least not then.

Insomnia kept me up the entire night. All I could think about was how to apply for a new passport to protect my identity, and because my mind is sharp, even without mania compounded on top of it, I soon had the answer.

While Yuni rested her eyes and tried to sleep, I couldn't enjoy the same. I kept thinking of ways, and opportunities, through which I could just leave Indonesia and take Yuni with me.

I knew I had to do something about this situation, and it was becoming increasingly difficult to do so with a mind on a rampage.

★ ★ ★

As day broke, I called my friend Wayan to ask him for a favor.

"Can you please send me a driver for the day?" I requested, knowing that I wouldn't have to say another word for him to help me.

When the driver, Ketut, arrived, he took Yuni and me to Finns, a beach bar in Berawa, where we sat and contemplated our next move.

"You seem really tense, Andy…" Yuni grazed the rough skin on my cheeks and smiled only slightly, "Care to take a walk with me?"

"Yes Yuni, soon" I agreed, knowing that I may feel more relaxed after a peaceful walk under the sun.

By now, Yuni knew that I had left all my documents in the safe in the room at Ibis Styles in Denpasar that I had paid for the day before and said we should go to get them. "No" I protested, "It's not safe, Yuni".

So instead, we asked Ketut to go to the hotel and pay for the room for an extra night. He must have been utterly confused why someone would pay for an empty room but he agreed nonetheless.

I insisted on not bribing the hotel staff and informed Ketut that I would only pay the exact amount I had paid for the room the day before. There was no way anyone would frame me for something - so I had to be careful about the minor things too.

After Ketut headed to Denpasar on his mission, Yuni and I went for a walk around Berawa, trying to be as normal as possible. We soon found a cafe with a pleasant garden at the end of a dead-end road.

By this point, I'd had an email from work agreeing to give me the week off. Looking around, I could see it was more than a cafe. It was also a collection of villas and it was a lovely spot.

I agreed to pay 13 million rupiahs for six nights which equated to around $930. I know, it was an absurd amount of money, but money was the least of my concerns. I figured I would claim it back from my company once all of the mess was over.

After all, they had to pay retribution for causing all of this!

It seemed like a viable option to rent a luxurious villa on a no-name basis and I told Yuni that it would be our safe place for the next little while. I would only be known as the 'sick guy' and it would strictly be only my family that could call me. As I put these demands to the staff, they cooperated with me and listened to every requirement dutifully.

That night, Yuni and I visited her aunt for dinner. It was a brave decision by her, knowing how I was acting and considering that I had never met her before. After the lovely meal, we took a taxi to Renon to meet my friend, Jero, who had been to Ibis Styles earlier to clear my room and the contents in the safe.

Yuni had, rightfully, convinced me at this point that it was crazy to pay for a hotel room on top of the villa. More importantly, she reminded me that I needed to get back on my medication, which I had left in the safe.

I listened to her because she wanted only what was best for me. She had also expressed her concerns about me not showing her enough affection. What she meant was that *I needed it,* rather than her.

When we returned to the villa in Berawa, we were exhausted. While lying on the sofa, I rested my head peacefully on her tummy and let her play with the strands of my hair. With every touch and embrace, I felt love and comfort in the only person I trusted – Yuni.

That night, I bawled my eyes out while lying with the woman who made me so comfortable with my vulnerability.

"I'm right here, Andy." She would whisper in her sweet, melodious voice. All I needed to hear then was just this, that she was right there with me.

Luckily enough, I could shed as many tears as it took to *finally* go to sleep.

Chapter 4: On the Run

After everything that had happened the night before, I was still awake early. That's what mania does to you. You're instantly on when you wake, no matter what time it is.

Immediately after waking up, I cleaned up the table and made it look tidier than ever. I hadn't realized what an odd activity that I had picked for myself until Yuni walked out of the room and stared at me.

"You don't normally do that" she commented rather suspiciously.

To be fair, I am a messy person. Cleaning the table was more of an impulsive itch than a chore that I would choose to do.

I can't recall if we had breakfast or not but I had a revelation that morning, that I had a son. The thought was madness, but I believed it.

Back in New Zealand, Mum had made friends with a university student from Saudi Arabia, and she always said that Ali looked like Dev Patel, the famous British

Indian actor. I knew Ali's age and somehow I figured he was my son from a one-night stand that I'd had in Kenya in 1999.

I told Yuni, and I am sure that she was utterly confused, but I was delighted at the thought of having a son. I deduced that Ali had contacted Mum to tell her his story in the hope she'd bring us together one day.

I was over the moon.

That morning, I went with Yuni to pick up her son from school. She then went to her house and put me in the taxi that would take me straight back to the safe place, the villa in Berawa.

As I made my way back, I felt as if complete serenity had embraced every inch of me - which was certainly quite eerie compared to what happened the night before. It was a feeling that I had never experienced before, being completely in sync with the world around me. My mood was in complete contrast to how it had been before, away from all the chaos and mess.

I was at peace, somehow, living normally until all the serenity finally came crashing around me.

The New Zealand consulate happened to be right next door to the villa. For some reason I decided to go in, and as I walked there, a horrible thought began feeding off me.

Could the consulate be 'in bed' with those who wanted to steal my identity?

Now, this was a fresh fear unlocked. I was absolutely spooked by all that my mind was making me think and believe.

Without thinking about anything else, I ran away from the consulate and saw a car waiting outside the villa. Fearing that someone was stalking me, I ran inside LV8, a hotel that I had known to be popular with Russians. The next thing I knew, I was at the reception and about to book a room because the villa no longer felt safe.

No matter which corner I sought refuge in, I would distrust a whole new person or organization.

'They're waiting for me!'

I couldn't help but revel in those feelings of paranoia, where I constantly believed that whoever the bad guys were, they would wait for me somewhere - eager to see which move I would make. My eyes went right toward the receptionist, as I noticed her talking on a walkie-talkie.

Perhaps she was talking to those people? Maybe they were waiting for me at the gate? For all I knew, the entire place could have been a trap, and I had walked right into it!

Without hesitating, I ran out the back door, desperate to get to the safety of the beach.

★ ★ ★

I set out to make my way south while staying close to the sea. I kept a wary eye out to ensure that I wasn't being followed. If I stuck close to other people walking on the beach, I could blend in with the crowd. Surely, I would be safe from anyone planning to shoot me with a sniper rifle?

However, some stretches of beach were empty. This forced me to run as fast as possible while in the sea, creating a new problem: my new iPhone got soaked with seawater. So even if I had a charger, which I didn't, there was a good chance it would not work.

I thought that if I stayed on the beach all day, I would eventually make it to Jimbaran, a place five miles south that Yuni and I had always wanted to visit. If I could do that, she would know where to find me. It might take her a while to work it out, but I had to ensure my safety.

As I made it past the Batu Belig and Seminyak beaches, I found a relatively safe place in Legian where there were plenty of tourists and, most importantly, Balinese people.

I'd had one close encounter en route. There had been a man on the beach that I believed was posing as a sunglasses salesman and I feared that he had a gun in his bag. However, I had managed to get to safety before he could get a shot at me.

As I came off the beach, I walked into a hotel and looked around to determine what level of safety it afforded me. I found a cupboard where I could hide if I needed to and saw that there were a few different ways out if I needed to run. And with that, I relaxed, sat by the pool, and took some time to decide what to do next.

At that moment, I treated myself to a beer, something I hadn't done for six months. It was around 2 pm, and I was desperate to get a message to Yuni.

She was still out there, unaware of whatever the hell was going on. Four hours had passed since our last contact.

She worked at a hotel in Kedungu an hour away, so I thought that if I could get a motorbike courier to get a written message to a restaurant close to her work, it would eventually reach her, and she would be safe. She'd be going out of her mind with worry about my sudden disappearance.

However, alas, I talked to some of the staff at the hotel when I was in Legian and, although they were friendly, they could not help me. With that, my suspicion rose tenfold, and I began overthinking the entire scenario again.

Why could no one see my crisis?

There was also a much simpler solution: I could have just used the hotel phone to call Yuni but, in my state of panic, the thought never entered my head.

In total shock, I took a walk for a while and was soon in the crowded shops of Kuta. I had been running around in the same clothes all day, and I thought that someone could recognize me now. I couldn't have that, so it was time to buy a new outfit. I went for a Bintang hat and a red Balinese shirt and kept walking, feeling pretty sure I was safe now.

However, these brief moments of safety didn't last long. It didn't take much for me to get alarmed when I'd turn around and find someone staring at me. I could feel that my safety was threatened, with every head turning around to look at me.

Eventually, I found my way to Siolam Hospital where I had seen Dr. Joy two days earlier. Across the road was a big shopping mall. I walked through the mall into the car park and decided that this would be a good pick-up point if I got in contact with Yuni or another friend.

From there, I started walking down a backstreet and thought about how I should just disappear. I thought back to LV8 and how I had run out the back door—I would have been caught on CCTV cameras, but I was sure that no one would have been able to positively identify me.

At least, I hoped so.

It was quiet on that backstreet, with my mind slowed down, that I walked down an alleyway for no real reason. I saw it was a dead-end, but I noticed a place called 'Rima's Salon,' which made my head spin again.

Rima, of course, was the name of my deceased wife.

Upon inspection, the place was closed, and I took this as a sign that all I had been thinking over the last few hours was right. This was the place where I needed to begin to lay the tracks of my disappearance, that of Andrew McLean.

Feeling even more agitated, I began thinking about where to dump my driving license and bank cards, which were all in my back pocket. I contemplated what to do with my phone and other valuables. And as I kept walking through the backstreets of Denpasar, I pondered what name to call myself.

What would be my new identity?

Who could I become?

Enough time had passed, and I needed a new disguise to accompany my newfound identity. I dumped my shirt and hat to wear just a pair of shorts as I thought of new ways to change my appearance. However, my cash was running low, and there was no way I would use an ATM to retrieve money as I feared it would trigger an alert to my whereabouts.

If this doesn't give you an idea of how deluded I had become, I don't know what will. Not only did I have to disappear to be safe, I believed that the bad guys, whoever they were, could track me based on using my UK bank card at a foreign ATM!

However, moving back to the matters at hand, I needed a hat, anything that would help me to be anonymous. As I meandered through many shops, none would sell me a hat for the 10,000 rupiahs I had left, around 70 cents.

By now, I was getting very close to the road that would take me to Jimbaran, where Yuni would find me. I knew no one down there, so it would be completely safe. Yet, something in me told me to stop, and by this time, I was getting tired from all the walking. So I headed into Kuta.

The day felt like a long and hopeless maze. A maze that had no way out.

I wasn't sure where I was going until I came across ACE Hardware and went inside to buy a phone charger that I paid for with my UK credit card using a false signature. I'm uncertain about what that would have done to help my situation, but there wasn't a lot of thorough reasoning behind anything I did that day.

By now, I had decided that my new identity was 'Tian Strauss,' a former South African rugby player. It's worth saying something about how I came up with the name; Tian is short for Christian, my manager at work, while Strauss is short for Andrew Strauss, a former England cricketer.

Smart, right?

I figured that once I had the new documents showing me as half Zimbabwean and half Austrian, the identity change would be complete. I had to think about my accent, but that could wait a while.

There were more pressing situations at hand.

Once outside ACE Hardware, I found an electricity point, and as I had feared, the seawater had killed the brand new iPhone that I had bought the day before—it was dead.

At this point, I realized that I needed somewhere to rest and sleep for the night.

As I arrived at the first hotel I saw, I felt uncomfortable when the manager started asking me too many questions for my liking, eventually causing an involuntary need to flee the place. Soon after, I was at a small hotel where a lovely young Balinese lady greeted me. What I liked about this place was the CCTV camera and I agreed to pay 600,000 rupiahs ($43) for a one-night stay.

However, my biggest concern was yet to be addressed. This did not solve the problem of a safe place for Yuni to meet me, and she still did not know where I was. At this point, I was starving. So, I went to the ATM and then to a restaurant to order a pizza.

I also ordered a beer as it felt okay, given the stress that I was under.

While sitting there waiting, I noticed many people looking at me, and wrongly, I assumed they were spies. Now that I look back at it, I realize they were ordinary people like your average Joe - just busy enjoying their night. However, I just could not kick the newfound habit of suspecting everyone.

There was absolutely no point in staying at a place where I felt threatened by everyone, especially if they made eye contact with me. I decided I should take my pizza as *bungkus* (a takeaway) after finishing my beer.

As I arrived at the hotel, six men were surrounding the receptionist. This did not look like a safe situation for me, as I kept thinking about what they could do at a family hotel. Thinking quickly on my feet, I threw the money for the room at the receptionist and told her that my girlfriend, Dayu Aryani, would come soon. That had been the waitress' name that had just served me pizza and beer.

My mind was still running wild with all the possibilities of this situation. Yunita Aryani was my girlfriend's full name, and the agent handling my work visa application was called Ayu. Somehow, I had convinced myself to believe that a random restaurant worker, Dayu, was also involved in this mess.

I know, it sounds like total madness.

Out of all this, I concluded that the room that I had booked could be used as a trap for Ayu, the evil agent, and Kumara, my boss that I no longer trusted. I wanted to ensure that they got trapped and caught on CCTV, not me.

However, there was a bigger issue playing on my mind.

Are there really six men at the hotel reception, or am I just seeing things?

It's so unlikely that in less than an hour since my first visit and seeing it as no different to any other hotel, that six men would arrive, begin speaking to the receptionist and wait for me. I can only conclude that I must have been hallucinating.

Was it the tiny dose of alcohol or the fear that's causing me to hallucinate?

I, unfortunately, didn't have the answer to that. Perhaps, it was just a side effect of the severe mania that caused that reaction?

It reminded me of a time in The Priory when five people entered my room, and I feared for my life. *Was that a hallucination as well?* It couldn't have been because I knew exactly who was in the room then, by name. Conversely, at that hotel in Kuta, all the men looked the same.

Is it a mirage of evil? Or, perhaps, they were there, but not as I saw them. Not figures of danger, just regular people minding their own business.

Anyway, with that out of the way, I was soon on the move again. Through the streets of Kuta, I was carrying my takeaway pizza when I passed a restaurant where a lovely Sumbawan girl greeted me; however, I wasn't compelled to enter because I didn't feel safe.

I didn't feel safe anywhere.

As I walked around, I wondered what could have triggered the six men at the hotel to come after me.

Was it because I tried to charge my phone?

Was it because I used my credit card at the hardware shop? Did the staff at ACE tip off the six men about me, and they were now following me everywhere in Kuta?

If six men could appear out of nowhere at a random hotel, how bad could this get for me?

I ditched the brand-new iPhone into a bush and began marching on without thinking twice about it. And it's not like it was cheap.

To where? I had no idea.

Just somewhere that I could finally feel at peace.

It was even terrifying to realize that I was now in a part of Bali where I didn't know anyone - for which I cursed myself.

Why hadn't I just headed straight to Ubud, where all my friends lived?

Why had I not just taken a taxi with some Balinese driver to reach a safe place quickly?

Why, oh why, am I making all these stupid decisions?

The questions in my head were never-ending. As I waged a mental war on myself, I came upon a major intersection and staked it out. One road was far too dark to walk down, and there was no way I was going to go back the way that I had just come from.

I went into Burger King to sit for a while and immediately saw two extremely tall and buff men, who I assumed were the Russians I had run away from earlier at LV8. Yet again, I bolted out of there with no intention of returning, and when I noticed that the police had also left their positions on the street corner, I realized I was on my own, yet again.

I was overtaken by paranoia and panic, and I desperately needed an escape route. The mania kept buzzing in my head, feeding adrenaline into my body, convincing me that there was something around any corner that could hurt me.

I had ruled out the road towards Kerobokan, where I lived, because I didn't know that road too well. I had two choices: get in a taxi or run to the petrol station where two poverty-stricken families were begging the people stopped at the traffic lights.

I stopped a taxi, requesting the driver's KTP (his Indonesian ID card), which ended up checking out, but I still couldn't convince myself to trust him. As I waited for the traffic lights to turn green, I slammed the taxi door shut and made a run for it across the road.

I sought refuge with two Balinese women and sat down with them. I offered them my leftover pizza and beer, after which I relaxed slightly.

I spent an hour resting there to figure out my next move. Even though Balinese women were people that I could trust, I knew my faith in them wouldn't last too long.

While I rested there, a car halted in close range to us, freaking me out. I began feeling the mania creep in again; was there a sniper in the backseat?

And, again, I was on the run.

I ran up Sunset Road towards Legian, looking for places to hide if I needed to. The road was quiet during this time, and I was sure that I wasn't being followed.

Even though the pressure was slightly off now, I was still very cautious of my surroundings. I could've rested near a pipe that I found under the bridge, but I kept thinking about Yuni and how I had to get back to her.

I was in a state of mania and as I now know, it makes me do the opposite of what is the right or best thing to do. I'm unsure if it's the same way for other people who suffer from bipolar disorder, but it's frightening for me to know what it did to me - what it actually turned me into.

When I entered the main street of Legian, I felt relatively safe. However, I soon became deeply suspicious of all the motorbike-taxi drivers from Grab passing by and waiting on the side of the road.

Grab had recently become an English-teaching client of mine and my contact there was a lady called Ayu from Jakarta, and even though it's a common name in Bali, I began associating her with the visa agent that had caused all my work-permit problems. I figured that the drivers of her company were out to get me as well.

Slowly, the web of enemies grew bigger and bigger.

Honestly, it must've been pure comedy for the drivers to see me duck, weave, and sometimes shout, "Get away!" whenever any of the drivers went past me. For them, I was just a crazy guy acting weirdly in a busy tourist area.

I came across a busy bar and thought about entering but I eventually decided against it because I did not want to be trapped with no escape route. Deciding to walk down a quiet street, I came across a hotel called The Mango Tree. I felt a wave of peace wash over me as I entered the reception, 'mango' being the nickname that I had had since I was at school.

When I think back, I still wonder why I didn't call Yuni at this point. However, I give myself the benefit of the doubt, knowing my mind couldn't stop racing – let alone make reasonable decisions.

After an hour of cleansing my mind, I rented a guesthouse across the street from The Mango Tree, under my assumed name, Tian Strauss. I desperately needed to lie down. However, I kept thinking about Yuni and how I had to reach her somehow; she must've been worried sick!

There I was, stumbling through the streets of Legian, and she couldn't have possibly imagined where I was. I departed the guesthouse but left the door unlocked and left a Mango Tree business card behind, since Yuni knew I also loved mango juice, along with a 500 rupiah coin, something that I knew would positively identify me if she were to make it to the guesthouse.

I also knew that Yuni and I had a safe room if we were ever in danger. We could go to this place if we wanted to seek refuge anytime in the future.

It was now 10 pm as a wave of tiredness hit me. It absolutely beats me when I wonder why I didn't just stay in the room that I had just paid for and rest. I was utterly exhausted, but the mania brought back the ability to just soldier on.

After finding a taxi driver from Karangasem, who said he belonged to the same family as the beggars I met earlier, I finally felt at ease and headed straight for Yuni's sister's place.

Why didn't I go straight to Yuni's house? I wish I had the answer to that question.

I was assuming that every Balinese person was safe, and Yuni's sister was married to a Balinese man named Gede, so it automatically became a safe option for me. I didn't have enough money to pay the driver upon reaching my destination, but I gave him my credit card as security, and he left me his business card. I promised him we would hire him as Yuni's family's driver, too.

Walking down the alleyway to Gede's place, I realized that everyone was asleep. For a while, I lay down behind the family temple, safe in the hands of God, yet I could not sleep.

Bearing in mind that Gede hardly knew me, I woke him up and told him I needed to get to Yuni's place.

He must have wondered what on earth I was doing, but he said nothing bad to me. He helped me in my state of panic, ordered a motorbike taxi for me, and paid for it as well.

The twenty-minute trip passed quickly. As I kept my head down, I was sure that I was not being followed. I got off at a convenience store near Yuni's place and then had an important thought—was her place being watched?

Proceeding with caution, I checked the street ahead of me, and there seemed to be a guy on the lookout, so I decided it was an unsafe area. I needed to lie low for a while. I made my way along the main street and lay in a ditch. In the distance, I could see a taxi that was not moving. Once it moved, I thought, I will too, but it stayed there for what seemed an eternity.

I looked at other options to escape, including an alleyway on the other side of the street, but I had no idea where it led, so I sat still. Maybe I could have fallen asleep there, but I was still wired and I was very close to Yuni's place.

It was probably around 3 am, and I had been awake since around 7 am. I was tired but also alert, and aware of everything happening in my surroundings.

As I lay there pondering my crazy day, I heard a sound that I liked, that of a stream of water, and I crawled towards it on my knees in a ditch. I then saw that a stream cut between the houses, and I was soon on my feet, knowing it led towards Yuni's house.

As I came to where the stream intersected the road, I looked left and right and saw no danger. So I crept quietly down the road and as I peered around the corner, I saw a motorbike with its lights on outside Yuni's compound. Feeling uneasy, I found refuge in an empty lot at the top of the street and laid down to rest.

I don't think I slept at all that night, and when the day broke, I made my move. With no obvious danger, I walked into Yuni's compound around 6 am. I'd never been inside before, I had only dropped her off, so I crept around as the residents started to wake trying to work out which was Yuni's door.

I talked to a lady called Nita, short for Yunita, like Yuni, and she was just lovely. She was from Sumatra, an island in the far west of Indonesia, but she had lived in Bali for many years with her Australian husband. She calmed me down and pointed me to Yuni's flat. She even suggested a company called Karma, where I might find work.

With that, I knocked on Yuni's door and we embraced and sat outside for a coffee to reflect on what had happened. She was relieved to see me but not as happy as I was to see her—thankful to know that she was alive and well.

It had been the single craziest day of my life.

Chapter 5: Getting to a Safe Place

It had been three days since Yuni had gone to work - because of me - and I knew she needed help in this situation. Now that I think about it, I realize she should've called Dr. Joy, who was best equipped to understand me in this hyperactive state of mania. Instead, we got in a taxi headed for After Taste, a cafe close to my apartment in Kerobokan, so that we could have breakfast.

As the taxi stopped outside, all I could see was a cafe full of Russians. None of the usual staff or customers were there. Maybe I was hallucinating again but it felt like another trap, so I told our driver to keep moving.

We eventually made it to the main road, at which point Yuni said we had to stop and pay the fare. As we got out next to a street market, all I could see were Muslim people. And while they were just going about their daily business, I rapidly descended into extreme paranoia.

At this point, I told Yuni to call Kadek, my friend in Ubud, to see if he could rescue us. All I wanted was a safe place, and Ubud was, in my mind, the best and obvious choice.

Kadek must have wondered why I was speaking the way I was, with the sound of desperation in my voice. At this point, Yuni took the phone and assured me everything would be okay. Except it wasn't.

My paranoia led us down the street next to Kerobokan jail and eventually to Sunset Road. Yuni complained of hunger pains, but I said that we needed to keep going until we found a cafe that I deemed to be safe.

Yuni then called Yani to tell her what was going on. I can only imagine how that conversation must have gone but I wasn't listening - I was on the lookout for the enemy.

As I was with Yuni, I felt at complete peace as we ate our food. After an hour, Yani arrived with her friend Joanna to collect us and take us to Ubud. I lay down on Yuni's lap in the back seat and tried to get some shut-eye. Yuni told Yani to first take us to the villa in Berawa so she could collect all my possessions.

While Yuni and Joanne went inside the villa to get my things, I peered outside the window to see if anyone was watching us. That was when I realized this was the exact spot where my crazy escapade the day before had first begun.

★ ★ ★

An hour later, Yani dropped us off at Kafe, a cafe in the center of Ubud, owned by Kadek, my friend I'd spoken to on the phone earlier. I couldn't have wished to be in a safer place, but I wondered why Kadek hadn't come to see me. After waiting a few hours, Yuni and I decided to rest at Yani's house.

I don't remember much about what happened next, but there was one terrifying thing. As they tried to put me to sleep on the sofa, and when Yuni left to go home, I could barely see her face. I knew it was indeed Yuni, but her face was blurred - just like the realities in my mind.

I'm pretty sure I was hallucinating again, and I can only assume that my illness was the culprit. I should've been in a hospital receiving medical care, yet here I was at my friend's house in Ubud, trying to make the best of a bad situation.

I fell asleep, but I woke up again at 1 am, which brought multiple epiphanies. This is normally what happens when mania hits me - I feel alert and always needing to be 'doing' something.

I began writing utterly incoherent words as I struggled to write legibly, but remarkably, I was soon writing with a precision that I had never managed before. I wrote with perfect handwriting, scribbling various notes with well-ordered numbering systems!

Between 1 am and daybreak, I wrote a lot to many people. It felt like my thoughts flowed endlessly, coming to me like revelations.

My mania seemed to work in a cycle of never-ending regrets. On Friday morning, I went for a walk and returned with the idea that I would resign from my English First job. With the letter drafted, full of demands and angry remarks, I showed it to Yani, who suggested I consult Yuni first.

However, I insisted I didn't need to. My god, I wish I had.

Clearly, my mind was spiraling out of control. Yuni was my girlfriend, and I needed to hear her opinion before doing anything drastic that could cause me harm in the future. Losing my job after The Priory 18 months earlier had catastrophic consequences, yet here I was, setting myself up for certain depression.

However, considering my mental state, it was difficult for anyone to reason with me. I feel like Kadek could've helped knock some sense into me if he had been there to do so, but he didn't appreciate how bad things were, nor would I have expected him to. Dad could've helped too, but he was in New Zealand preparing to travel to France for a holiday and he had no idea about my full-blown psychosis.

I promised Yani that I would return to her house after posting my resignation letter at the post office. It turned out that the post office did not provide same-day deliveries to Denpasar, and it being a Friday, I wanted the letter to arrive at English First before the weekend.

Eventually, I found my way to Kafe, where I had been with Yuni the day before. I requested a security guard to help me in my quest to get the resignation letter to Denpasar, and went inside to order a coffee and wait.

As I looked around after waiting a few minutes, I noticed a different man approaching me. I immediately became suspicious of the man and went outside to find the security guard, who had also magically disappeared.

Then, as if on impulse, the ringing alarm bells in my head began making me paranoid once more. Beginning to freak out, I ran out of the back door of Kafe and found my way to Kadek's house upstairs.

Such was my luck, though. Kadek was not home, and my paranoia was quickly getting the better of me. I noticed his cleaner and began berating her, learning that she had worked for Kadek for six months. I demanded that she let me use the phone, after which I called Yani, who said that my friend, Jero, would come to pick me up in ten minutes. Clearly, they were both really worried about me being on my own.

Anxious and afraid, I waited on the front steps of Kadek's house, desperately hoping that Jero would arrive before something else began making me paranoid and sending me off on the run. Upon Jero's arrival, we got on her motorbike and went to my friend's *warung* (a small restaurant), where she forced me to eat something.

I began asking Jero ridiculous questions such as "Is it normal for a Muslim woman to work at the post office?"

Jero reminded me, "Yes. Not everyone is out to get you, Andy."

But maybe, they were.

I hadn't forgotten about my resignation, though. I was determined to do what I had planned, and as soon as Jero took me back to Yani's house, I emailed work with my letter of resignation. I did the unthinkable - something done without considering the dire consequences for my mental well-being.

After resigning, I would be unemployed in a place where it was almost impossible to find regular employment. I didn't think about anything! I didn't think about how irresponsible I was for not valuing my welfare over all these thoughts running through my mind.

Don't assume I did not love my job, I did. However, my psychosis wasn't allowing me to think straight or comprehend even the basic situations of life. At that moment, when I pushed send on the email,

I didn't care what it meant for me in the future. I just wanted to finish it as soon as possible because I distrusted my company.

I just wanted a break. With that, I went back to sleep for the rest of the afternoon.

★ ★ ★

When I opened my eyes, the entire place was dark, and no one was at Yani's house.

Why had my friends left me alone?

I assumed it was to make me feel that I was safe at Yani's place.

Indeed, as I walked outside of the house and looked around, I felt at peace. Maybe, I was safe here. However, where did they go? I was curious about their whereabouts and I walked down the path to search for where they could be.

Maybe they are at the restaurant nearby, waiting for me?

I walked and walked, but there was no sign of anyone in all the obvious places to look for them. I knew the area well and found my way around, landing at a big restaurant complex I had never been inside of.

Wandering, I reached a place where some people were having a party. However, despite none of my friends being there, I convinced myself to believe it was a reception party for me. A staff member handed me a beer, and I sat by the water, feeling at peace as I waited for my friends to arrive.

My eyes met those of a few other people sitting some tables away from me, who looked like they were from China.

Were these my students, the ones I taught online? Had they come to see me?

I tried my best to stop my mind from running wild again. Feeling agitated as I waited, I walked upstairs and came across some Balinese outfits.

These must be for Yuni and me. There was to be a big party celebrating our relationship.

However, with no guests of mine approaching the restaurant, I concluded that the party must be tomorrow instead of today. Maybe this was all a grand gesture to make me feel safe again, and perhaps, my entire ordeal might be over soon.

One can only hope, my friend.

With that thought, I exited the restaurant and returned to Yani's house. Walking along the road, I saw the word 'Lekker' written on a shop sign, which I immediately began associating with the South African bank that I used to work for in London.

Maybe my old colleagues were also in town for the party?

I wanted to tell my friends about everything I had seen but had no phone. Upon returning to Yani's house, I was so tired from all my walking and thinking. Exhausted and frustrated, I soon fell asleep again.

Chapter 6: Discovering
that I was a Secret Agent

Whenever you see someone in a state of mania or psychosis, the best thing to do is seek medical help.

However, with no one understanding what was going on with me, and I was in no state to realize that I was out of control, I didn't receive the medical attention I desperately needed. I kept living my life the way normal people do, in the most abnormal ways.

I decided I wanted to return to my apartment in Kerobokan, the one I had deemed unsafe a couple of days ago. It would also mean being close to Yuni who, by now, was having a well-deserved break from me while trying to maintain her job and family life.

I can't recall how I got back to Kerobokan, but it was a Saturday night and Yuni and I went to Gapet, our favorite restaurant, to have dinner. At this point, my psychosis reached even more absurd heights.

After having some food, the owner, Albert, came to sit down and chat with us. We knew him well from many previous visits, and I was not suspicious of him. However, as we sat there, I felt a revelation in my mind. I'm unaware of how I received it, but I now knew I was a secret agent.

Remember that I never received a formal message, written or otherwise, but this revelation was a vivid experience.

In essence, I had just been told that my family were secret agents, somehow involved in a plot to bring down corrupt oil companies. The details were sketchy, but they somehow related to when my grandfather worked for Mobil Oil and the real reason my family had lived in the Chatham Islands, 300 km east of New Zealand, when I was a young boy.

And now that my mission was revealed, I knew that I was supposed to be taking the lead in setting up a bank on the island of Bali. I'm not sure how this was linked to the oil scandal, but it did not matter.

I quickly took out a piece of paper and pen, writing down how I'd work with this elaborate scheme and who would be included in it. It only took me a couple of minutes to figure out the entire plan, mainly because all the people involved were friends of mine at Investec, the bank that I had worked for in London.

Please bear with me, for it will all make sense later.

As I returned to the table with my plan and showed it to Yuni, I realized that Albert must've also seen it and this was now a top-secret matter. I tore the plan up and we promptly left Gapet and started walking back to my apartment.

At that moment, I began thinking that Yuni was also a secret agent, but I didn't know how she was involved. However, that didn't help the deep suspicion that I had about her in my mind, even though she was my girlfriend and I shouldn't have expected such a thing from her. And, of course, she had no idea of what was going through my mind.

As we walked down the quiet street, I had a sudden, random thought: *when was my next doctor's appointment?*

I immediately called Dr. Joy, demanding, "You should've told me why I have been hallucinating. You should've told me that I was susceptible to it!"

It was around 8pm on a Saturday night, and I could hear Dr. Joy's kids in the background - I'm sure she wasn't expecting my call, and that too with such shocking news. However, she handled the call well and agreed with the criticism, saying, "Okay, Andy. Let's meet on Monday to discuss your condition better."

I told Dr. Joy that I was, unjustifiably, concerned about the little white pill she had prescribed earlier in the week. To me, it felt like it was the reason I was hallucinating, which is why I demanded answers from her.

As I later discussed with her, I was so manic about what was going on at work that when I saw her, I didn't do what I always did – ask exactly what she was prescribing and what it was for.

When Yuni and I returned to my apartment, I was so disoriented by the entire situation that I decided to take the piss out of it, quite literally. Perhaps, I was so distraught with my family for not informing me I was a secret agent.

Because of my new suspicion of Yuni, I demanded that she sit on a chair in front of the CCTV cameras as I sat in front of her. I interviewed her, completely naked, and she just sat there, smiling.

I didn't even know what I was interviewing her about.

While this was happening, Niko, a fellow resident in the block, stopped by and I grabbed a chair for him to be interviewed also. I'm unsure who I was trying to broadcast the entire thing to, but Niko was surprised at my demand. He said, "Whatever you're taking, I want some of it."

Thus, the interview rambled on for a while.

I guess Niko just believed I was interrogating them for fun, while Yuni must have been delighted to have someone else present to work out what to do with me.

That Saturday night, Yuni only slept a few hours and she told me that she was 'unsure' of me. In reality, the only thing we could be sure of was that 'whatever I was on' totally fucked me over the next day.

Chapter 7: The Great Heist

On Sunday morning, when I woke up early, I was immediately pressed with another appalling situation.

What if my apartment is being haunted by evil spirits?

With this thought, I began taking things out of my room and laying them out on the balcony. I believed that was how I could cleanse my room of any ill will I had been associating myself with.

Why would I entertain such thoughts, you might wonder?

It's quite simple for a bipolar mind to come to conclusions because of the rummaging mess in the boundaries of our skull. I still had my late wife's suicide note from 2012, and I was sure it needed to go. It had hung over me for way too long. I also took out my uniform as a teacher at English First, since work was another huge source of evil in my life.

I know how you must be laughing at the condition of my mind. Perhaps, you might be relating as well.

At that moment, Yuni woke up and questioned my behavior.

"You shouldn't keep your things outside, even if you're planning to cleanse your room." Yuni had tried to convince me, "It's all getting moved outside your neighbor's door, and you know how she is."

It is worth saying something about my neighbor, a lady from Russia. I had never spoken to her, but she habitually complained about me. It turns out that she had also complained about Catherine, my other neighbor from Sulawesi.

She had been rude and abrupt to me in the past, never bothering to speak with a little decency. However, by now, she had become mildly friendly – she started acknowledging me as a human being.

That morning, I concluded she was also a secret agent, part of the entire plot. I did not sense any immediate danger from her so I assumed I was safe for the time being.

It's also worth mentioning Catherine at this point. She had been staying in the room next to mine, and we got on well. She was a beautiful young woman, much younger than Yuni and she never acknowledged Yuni.

By this time, she had moved out and her apartment was empty, which led me to have yet another crazy thought.

Had she been planted there to see if I would cheat on Yuni?

I was sure she had been, even if she had never made an advance at me. So I gave myself a pat on the back to have passed this test to prove that Yuni was the one for me, the woman that I would soon marry.

That Sunday morning, I began working on cracking the code. I know, I know, what code, right? I didn't even know how this had become part of my mission, or why it was even given to me. Honestly, I can't even remember what 'cracking the code' meant!

All I knew at that moment was that it was my task to do and, from here, the story gets even more perverse.

I sat outside my apartment with a notebook, working through the clues as they appeared. Every time I took a break or spoke to Yuni, another clue appeared when I got back to my seat.

What if it's the Russian lady leaving clues for me? Or could it be Niko as well, the guy who lives a few doors down?

It's impossible to describe what I was doing because I didn't keep that notebook. Everything that ran through my head was hasty and hazy. All I know is that I was methodically working through what I thought were 'clues'.

And still, I was quite unsure of what it all meant.

I worked out a safe zone in the triangle shape of a yacht's sail, extending from Ubud in the north to Denpasar airport in the south, to Kedungu in the west. With this knowledge, the unsafe place was Kuta, although I already knew that from my day on the run around a couple of days before.

It was around 11 am when Yuni made us breakfast because she knew I needed some energy to keep me going. I thought, incorrectly, that Yuni knew *exactly* what was going on. I was certain she was also a secret agent working with me. I had assumed we were on this mission together, and though I never spoke to her directly about what I had been doing, I assumed she was privy to the task I had been given.

As we ate our eggs, I talked to Yuni about 'cracking the code' and showed her what I had figured out. I showed her the map of Bali that I had drawn and asked her to point to Ubud.

She stared at me with a befuddled look, and I'm sure she must have wondered what the point of it all was as she had lived in Bali for twenty years. But, she said nothing, so I again assumed that we were both on the same page and that she had a role to play in all of this craziness.

While my thought process was a little chaotic, I found some reasoning behind my actions. I had assumed that people I knew were working on an elaborate plan that had been manifesting into existence for a long time. I reasoned that this dated back to when my grandfather worked for Mobil Oil in New Zealand.

I can say one thing, and that is my affirmation that there were some wrongs in the past that my family had been involved in. One thing led to another, and I believed that I had to devise a plan to right the wrongs of the past, which had many facets to them.

Nelson Mandela's quote helped reorient my choice, "As long as poverty, injustice, and gross inequality persist in our world, none of us can truly rest."

I, for one, was not interested in any rest.

Not that I was getting any, that is.

Amid my mania, I firmly believed that the 'bad guys' were to end up in the gas chambers of Auschwitz, those from World War Two that I had once visited many years earlier. The world's riches were to end up in Bali at UOB Bank. After that, my task would be to distribute funds to rid the world of poverty.

This all made perfect sense to me as, although Bali is a Hindu island in a Muslim country, it's known as the Island of the Gods. It's also located near the equator which, for some reason, I thought was significant.

UOB is a Singaporean bank with operations in Bali, and my placement there as a teacher over the previous few months had come via English First. In other words, I had been planted at English First to gather intelligence for the secret mission I was now on.

This led me to assume that English First was not my enemy, but it was still involved in the plot in some way. Others were involved too.

I somehow deduced that the hotel where Yuni worked in Kedungu was a hoax and that the reason that it had not opened yet was not because it was not ready to open but because it was involved in the plot. My starting assumption was that its owners were siding with the 'bad guys,' even though I had not yet figured out who exactly these people were.

The more I thought about it, the more I believed that the owners of Yuni's hotel were crooks involved in the plot and that the hotel was a cover for some sort of illegal activity. But, I did not doubt Yuni—she was merely a pawn in a messy game, albeit one related to her being a secret agent. I felt that she had been put there for a reason other than being the HR Manager.

However, there was one odd thing; Yuni's hotel was inside the safe zone, according to the map I had drawn. Hence, I could not attach any significance to that thought. This added to the confusion on the most bizarre day of my life.

★ ★ ★

I'm sure you must be interested in discovering how my family is even involved. However, bear with me, for I will reveal everything in good time. This brings me to my family's involvement and my old boss, Chris, back in London. The only connection between them was me, because my family and Chris had never met nor spoken to each other.

Yet, I was now convinced that Chris was, in fact, my brother, and that he had been working as a secret agent all his life. Before I was born, Mum had given a baby up for adoption and now, all these years later, I assumed that baby was Chris.

There are plenty of reasons why I believed that this was the case, but that's a story for another time. For now, just notice the way my mind connects dots, bringing forth evidence even though there may be nothing deducible.

Chris was raised in South Africa and was a senior manager at Investec in London. Being the brother I never had, I somehow concluded that his mission as a secret agent had been to rid the organization of evil, basically siding with the good guys, the Jews, in the company, rather than the majority non-Jews. This group included Jamie, who I have mentioned before, and James, who had visited me at The Priory.

Yet, despite all the positive signs, something inside me drove my mind into a deluded place. Chris couldn't be trusted.

By now, I had realized that Dad and Chris had hatched a plan to somehow intercept a huge amount of the world's riches and stash them on an island in Fiji, where Dad's yacht had been shipwrecked two years earlier. I also believed that it was Chris who wanted to steal my identity and move from London to New Zealand, where his wife's family lived.

I was livid, and with all these thoughts swirling around my head, I had to work out which side would get the money, even if I didn't really understand yet who each side was. All I knew was that a plot, which had been planned for decades, had come down to this moment.

I figured the plot had been planned after World War Two in such a way that the money would move around the world by ship to get to its final destination in Bali. But in the year 2019, funds could flow at the push of a button!

Trust me, I laughed at how ridiculous it all was, but I had a decision to make. Only one side would get their hands on the world's riches and, in my mind, it came down to a simple decision of choosing between *red* and *blue*.

For me, red represented good, while blue was bad. This was because red signified Liverpool, my favorite football team, and represented the Labour Party in the UK and New Zealand. Blue was the National Party in New Zealand, which all my family and friends voted for, and the Conservative Party in the UK.

I thought about what some other people that I liked would do and what would be best for the world – such as China becoming a superpower and Donald Trump trying to befriend North Korea.

Everything was pointing towards red, and my mind was made up. Yet, I still couldn't fathom why it was me that was having to make a decision that would have effects that would reverberate around the world for a long time to come.

Team Red would be the winner, but I was unsure what I needed to do with this information. Amid this mental ruckus, I had another problem to contend with, and I have no idea how this came about.

Since I had become the one chosen as the arbiter of this crazy situation with major international importance and my exact location was known, I now felt a huge amount of danger around me and felt far from safe. Yuni had been so quiet all morning, so I even doubted whether or not she was really on my side.

★ ★ ★

It had got into my head that we could be attacked at any moment, from any angle, so I told Yuni to stay inside while I kept watch outside. In doing so, I saw what appeared to be a helicopter hovering in the distance and assumed it had guns pointed directly at my apartment.

Now, I had to work out the angles at which we would be safe and where we could be hit. If a shot was to be fired, and I assumed it could be, I would take the bullet - not Yuni. I ran inside and held Yuni close, telling her not to move until I said so. I was certain that we could both be shot, and I got off the floor to position myself in front of her.

As I looked up, I could still see the helicopter in the distance, and I moved us to an angle where we were safe, and the pressure was off momentarily—we had survived. We couldn't relax yet, but the danger had been averted for the time being.

I'm sure that, at this point, I had freaked Yuni out as well. However, in my mind, I kept thinking that she was already aware of this situation we were in and she didn't need to be confused or scared.

I assumed that the helicopter must have disappeared. Regardless, I felt there was nothing more I could do.

At this moment, I also realized that 'cracking the code' was irrelevant—because if I did nothing, there would be no winners and losers. It was a truly bizarre feeling.

Almost arbitrarily, I decided my mission was complete. *The Great Heist* was over!

There would be no winner because I had not given the code to either side.

Team Blue, which Dad, Chris, and all my friends were on, had lost because I did not trust their motives and I had felt that they had totally misjudged me. Team Red, including my friends at Investec, James and Jamie, had not won either.

I didn't understand why I was 'the chosen one' for this mission but I was certain that this situation of being a secret agent was something I did not like. Perhaps, this was the point of it all; that I was chosen for a reason.

Maybe I was not meant to choose a side at all.

Maybe I was meant to hand over the responsibility to something greater than myself.

Maybe I was meant to hand over the responsibility to God.

But, why the hell had I been put in this position? Out of every other person on the planet, why me?

More worryingly, I felt that by determining that there would be no winner, I had inadvertently put Yuni and I in danger. By not choosing a side, both sides were now livid and I concluded that if one of us had to be sacrificed, it should be me.

In the early afternoon, Yuni said that she needed to do her weekly grocery shopping. Perplexed, I explained that this felt like a reckless decision.

I was certain that she would be a target if she left my apartment. Yuni was definitely conflicted about what she should do but she had to make sure her family was okay, even though she was really worried about me too.

I understood her decision to leave, even though I was initially upset. I looked at Yuni with my eyes full of love and adoration, as I smiled with a heavy heart, "Go home, love. You need to be safe with your son and mum. Leave me be. I'm old enough to take care of myself."

I walked with her to the end of the street and apologized to her for abandoning her – it was safer for her if I stayed at my apartment. I promised to do my best to make it to her birthday dinner on June 3rd, in a week's time.

"I love you, dear Yuni." I caressed her cheek, leaving a soft kiss as I continued, "I'll see you soon."

She waved at me as she walked into the distance, and I waved back.

My heart dropped as I wondered when I would see her again, or if I would be blessed enough to actually see her at all.

Chapter 8: The Calm Before the Storm

It was now the late afternoon of Sunday, May 26th, 2019 as I walked back to my apartment, reflecting on the enormity of what had happened that morning. I literally had a gun to my head, albeit from a helicopter far off in the distance.

Yet, somehow, I had averted the danger. How? I wasn't sure. Maybe I was just a lucky man.

However, things like this do not happen to people who are 'lucky.'

It was probably around this time I thought about the people I admired: Mandela, Mahatma Gandhi, Richard Branson, and the Dalai Lama. All people who took no sides. I felt a deep admiration and connection to these people, as I could now understand the strife that comes with that way of life.

I felt vulnerable but relieved to be in the *safe triangle* of Bali.

However, I felt anger boiling within me, sending heat throughout my body. I was beyond irate at some of my family members —my sister, Rebecca, Dad, and my uncle, David. I figured they had all played a part in *The Great Heist* and duped me.

Still, I had reserved my biggest resentment for David. Who is David, you may ask?

David is the brother of my late step-grandmother, Brenda. This makes him the uncle of Brenda's son, Scott, who visited Mum, Dad, and me in the Chatham Islands when we lived there.

Scott gets another fleeting mention in this story, whereas David is about to become a significant character in it.

You see, David could have rescued me from The Priory's hellhole when he visited me there and I was living in fear. However, since he was so swooned by a nurse, one that I didn't trust with my care, it felt to me that he wasn't trying to understand what I was going through.

Since I was in a state of mania, my words of retaliation mattered very little. Naturally, I resented David and my mates, Nick and Rob, for leaving the hospital to have a beer instead of petitioning to get me out of there.

I'm sure they believed that they were relying upon the best information they had but it is also important to listen to the patient as well. The patient may complain about something that feels very real, yet those that aren't privy to what happens 'on the inside' might just think of those complaints as the sounds flies make when they buzz over their ears.

Annoying and pointless.

While this crazy episode was unfolding in Bali 18 months later, Dad had traveled to meet David in France to look for a fancy yacht to buy.

Now I knew why. They had wanted to profit from *The Great Heist*.

"Fuck them," I thought, "They're definitely going down."

By late afternoon, I felt ecstatic for having broken this code of utter nonsense, put together by some of the world's most brilliant minds. However, lingering in the back of my mind was the thought that if I had chosen to pick a side, I could have potentially saved the world from the corruption that would reign for the rest of our lives.

Corruption that my family was directly involved in.

At some point, Niko, my neighbor, came to see me because he was worried about how I was doing. I don't quite recall the question he asked me, but I remember it was an innocent one, one that led me to assume that he, too, was a secret agent.

As I talked to Niko about what had happened that morning, I felt as if he was also somehow connected to the entire thing. I said that I should be compensated for what I had gone through. He must have wondered what on earth I was on about but, nonetheless, he agreed with me.

After Niko left, I walked to Gapet, the restaurant up the road where I had been with Yuni and Albert the night before. I had a feeling of pure elation at cracking the code. I sat down at the table closest to the Balinese temple, so that I would have God's protection, and ordered a beer—I felt that I had earned it. And, as I gazed out across the Gapet lawn, I saw lots of kids dancing and playing.

I was a long-term customer of Gapet and had seen nothing like this —it was often just Yuni and I there. Today though, it must have been a celebration of the world having been freed of poverty and corruption. It was the utopia that the world had been waiting for. The scenes of jubilation were amazing to see.

This was the hard evidence that I needed to confirm that my mission had been worth it.

I asked the waiter to get a message to Yuni, who lived around three kilometers away. I gave the basic location, close to a petrol station, and figured the people who worked there would know where she lived. At this point, my delusions were in overdrive.

Would Gapet's staff really send someone to find Yuni and, second, would they be able to find her?

While it was an unlikely scenario, I sat there and began thinking of the culprits in this mess.

I pointed to a packet of cigarettes, Yuni's favorites, towards the infamous Kerobokan jail which was just a stone's throw away. After that, I ordered another beer, one of three or four that I had that night.

I decided that the people who would go to jail would be my sister, Rebecca, but only long enough for her to 'wake up' to be a better daughter and mother, along with Dad, Chris and David. They all deserved to be in jail for what they had done to me.

With Chris, after doing time in Kerobokan, he would be sent to Robben Island in South Africa, the country he had grown up in where Mandela had spent twenty-seven years incarcerated; David would spend time in Belmarsh in England, while Dad would serve all his time in Kerobokan jail.

Seeing all the celebrations of a free world around me, I felt I had done my job. I was forty-four years old and I'd never had an inkling that I was, in fact, a secret agent, but I had carried out my mission.

If some of my family members were to go down as a result, so be it.

Soon after this, Yuni arrived with my friend, Jero. She didn't come because the waiter had asked her to, but simply because she was seriously worried about me and had enlisted the support of Jero to come see me.

Yuni always knew where to find me—at Gapet.

When they arrived, I outlined my plan to put my family in jail. They seemed to agree with me, but their primary goal was to get me to a safe place to sleep peacefully and rest. I also began writing a series of notes I asked Yuni to send Rebecca via What's App.

Honestly, it must have been a truly bizarre experience for Rebecca to receive what she did.

One note said 'no more yachts,' while another said 'and don't interrupt my dinner again,' a reference to the previous night when I had first received the message that I was a secret agent. That was important because it was the six-month anniversary of my relationship with Yuni. And most bizarrely of all, I wrote a demand that Chris, Rebecca, David and Scott meet in the Chatham Islands to sort the mess out, whatever that meant.

And I said they had only forty-five minutes to devise a solution.

It was around midnight New Zealand time when Yuni sent the messages, so Rebecca would not have received them until she woke in the morning. And when she did, she would have been on high alert that something was seriously wrong with me.

For some reason, I took my food as a takeaway, and soon Yuni and I were alone again at my apartment as Jero went home to Ubub. What I really needed was both Yuni and Jero to put me to sleep but that did not happen and, soon, things spiraled out of control.

Chapter 9: The Night from Hell

My nerves were a wreck as I kept thinking about my family and all the harm they had caused me during this mission.

For some bizarre reason I began to quiz Yuni about her father, who had died some years earlier. I even suggested that Kadek was her real father, resulting from an affair he had had with her mum. The look of shock on her face stunned me and, of course, she denied it.

I don't have a good memory of what happened next, but I believe she shifted the power dynamics in our relationship as she sternly demanded, "Sit down, now, Andy. Just sit."

I listened to her. At that moment, her sentence made me shut up, despite the mania raging within me. Yuni is a petite woman, so this moment was powerful—she held power, and I knew it.

However, the moment did not last as I became obsessed about what would happen to me. I had gone from elated to extremely fearful and Yuni became the object of my anger fueled by fear.

I yelled at her, pleading, "Please, just help me. Don't you know how to help me?!"

Of course, she could do nothing even if she knew what I meant by 'help me'. Yuni simply froze, and I still remember the look of terror on her face. She sat there on the bed, helpless, and her eyes were like ice. It was an image I will never forget and one that I never want to see again. It pains me to write these words because she did not deserve the treatment she suffered from me that night.

But, because she couldn't or wouldn't help me, the anger turned into an ugly emotion that I don't wish to recall but I will, for the account of this book. My anger soon became violent as I hurled my dinner across the room in her direction and started kicking over the chairs outside.

Yuni curled up in a ball on the bed, most likely sobbing and praying for it all to end. I sat down outside, and as I pondered what to do, my thoughts became morbid—I decided that either Yuni or I would have to die if we didn't protect ourselves.

I went back inside the room, told her of my thoughts, and begged her to make some suggestions about how to resolve the situation, and eventually, she wrote some ideas in my notebook.

Finally, we are making some progress.

Yuni is such a calm person, and even though I had just terrorized her, she could still focus. She showed amazing resilience that night when really she should have just run away at the first available opportunity.

Instead of leaving me and running for her life, Yuni put me to bed and immediately began calling people. She called my friend, Tim, who happened to be in Australia rather than Bali, who urged her to ask someone from my family to come to Bali urgently. I have not asked Yuni if she slept that night, but I doubt she did.

If there is a hero in this story, it's her—despite being under immense pressure, she never wavered in her support for me. And she was spending nights away from her son and mum.

When I woke up the following morning, the first image I saw was of my friend, Candice, sitting outside my room. However, the rage in my mind hadn't subsided. As I looked at Candice's face, all I could see was Rebecca.

According to Candice, I spoke for forty-five minutes without letting her speak, which Yuni has also confirmed. She told me I was rude and aggressive, as well as criticizing her for why she was struggling with her business.

I don't remember it this way; it was a much shorter conversation for me. But I remember thinking that it was as if I was talking to Rebecca as Candice would not listen to what I had to say. This is the best explanation I can give of my bipolar mind at that moment, which distorted my grasp over reality.

Once I was finished with my tirade, I got up and let Yuni take over. I began sweeping the floor on the balcony and then went to a shop across the road and had a cigarette to calm down.

I went back to my apartment as Candice was getting ready to leave. I told her that I had forgiven the debt of $250, which she owed me from a week earlier, because she had come to my rescue that morning, and that I was grateful for that. Someone had to set me straight, and I was glad Candice could help Yuni.

Soon after this, Yuni left me to go to work. She had hardly been in the office for the past week, and in a moment of madness, I had kicked her work phone off the balcony and shattered it.

All she could say was "Why did you do that?" and as much as I tried to explain that her company was part of this evil plot, I'm sure she was just keen to get the hell out of there.

I was on my own for the rest of that day. I soon became lost in my thoughts, the most important of which was to work out who my new family would be.

Chapter 10: Accepting My New Life as a Secret Agent

Since it had now been confirmed that I was a secret agent, I knew that my life in the future would be radically different from what it had been in the past.

For starters, Dad and Rebecca would soon be in Kerobokan jail. But more than that, I realized that, as a secret agent, I was no longer in control of my life. Maybe, as Kadek once said to me, life had already been set out for me and I had no influence over the path it would take.

So, I thought through the consequences of what had just happened. Clearly, Mum was still my mum, and Sam was still my brother—that much I could be sure of, but the rest was a big question mark.

Kadek and Dad share the same birthday, so I assumed with the new identity I was about to have, that Kadek would now be my father. I also assumed that Jamie, my best friend at my old company in London, would become a new brother based in Bali, where we would soon set up a new bank.

I wasn't sure where this left Sam, but I knew that
Candice would replace Rebecca as my sister. Candice
is Canadian, about the same age as Rebecca, so there
were many ways for that part of the story to work.

However, I could not contemplate the loss of my Dad.
It became an overriding emotion, one that aggravated
me beyond comprehension. For forty-three years,
I had been his son, and I did not want to lose him.
However, I thought 'it is what it is' and I realized that
I simply had to deal with whatever trauma I would
face. After all, I was a secret agent, and there was no
way of opting out.

I didn't choose this life for myself, so I didn't get to call
any of the shots.

With all of this now apparent, things made sense, and
I knew why I was chosen for this job. This is when
another extreme thought burned inside my mind.

As the day passed, I pondered what life as a secret
agent would be like. I thought of James Bond, Sam's
favorite film character.

At some point, I got a message asking me what sort of
next mission I wanted. When I received it, I was in
my bathroom, and, as best I can remember, it involved
diving, and I said "No" immediately because I did not
feel fit enough for that type of challenge.

It was then that I came to believe that my apartment
had cameras in it, even if I couldn't see them, with

every move that I made being watched, every word being heard. And I began talking to whoever was listening, expressing my thoughts as they came to me.

In the safety of my bathroom, I was put through my paces to get an idea of how fit I was. I did a lot of running on the spot and concluded, especially after my day on the run the previous week, that I was quite fit despite becoming a smoker again two years ago.

What happened next was truly odd. I sat on the toilet, wiping my bottom, and blood appeared on the toilet paper.

This was not a surprise as I had an infection but what was weird was how I methodically laid the pieces of paper out on the floor until there was no blood left. I felt that leaving evidence of this infection was important. I wish I could explain why I did such a thing, but I have no words.

Eventually, I realized there were different options: to disappear immediately on a new mission or take some time out before being assigned my next mission.

As I pondered these options in the bathroom, I thought about what I needed to take with me and what would have to stay behind as evidence of someone having lived there for the next secret agent that would arrive.

I also scoped out the bathroom to ensure what worked and what didn't. One light didn't work, and I made a mental note for later. Perhaps, in the back of my mind, doing so clarified my bizarre situation – I needed to be sure that nothing would come as a surprise.

I methodically worked through the room, placing clothes on my bed that I might need to take if I had to leave quickly and generally securing the apartment. I also had to find what clothes were plain enough so they wouldn't identify me. For example, many of my t-shirts held significance to a certain date and place. As my next outfit, I settled on jeans and a plain white shirt, signifying peace.

I thought of my lost years and what this new life as a secret agent would afford me. I thought about losing Yuni. I thought that it would be okay, that it was part of the game that I had suddenly found myself in. Eventually, I concluded that I needed some time to think and told whoever was listening that I needed a break for a few hours to make my decision.

My mind was scrambled. Nothing was making sense.

I left my room and walked the short distance to After Taste, the cafe that I had driven past with Yuni the previous week, where I had hallucinated. On the way, I passed a small shop owned by a Muslim couple and pondered its significance. I had been going to the shop every day for three months and had looked at one of the rooms they rented out—I'd thought that I might need to stay there if Mum came to stay with me one day as my apartment only had one bed.

No one was around; the streets were quiet, bringing a sense of serenity to my otherwise overwhelmed mind. I sat in the cafe, ordered some food, and began thinking. Although I did not know what another type of mission might be, I figured out that my life could be erased from any point in its history.

For example, I could have a new story written for me from age eight, the age when I was truly happy and carefree, if that's what I wanted. I could have my entire life wiped out, or I could accept it for what it was and start afresh from age forty-three with a new identity.

None of this makes any sense as I write it now, but these were the thoughts that I had that afternoon. For a fleeting moment, I considered starting from the beginning, back in the Chatham Islands where I'd lived when I was one and two years old, but that came with one major drawback—it was a certainty that I would lose Yuni and, most likely, my family.

In the end, I somehow came up with a four-year mission because I felt I had lost four years of my life since 2015. In other words, the clock would rewind four years, erasing those four years of my life.

That four-year period had been harrowing for me, with long periods of unemployment, no place to call home, and considerable depression. It seemed a fair ask to be compensated for the situation I now found myself in as a secret agent.

I also reasoned that my new mission could be in Bali, and that I would get to choose what it would be. It could be setting up the new bank, but it didn't have to be—whatever the case, I decided I would be the one to set the terms of my next deployment.

I wanted to ensure that I could still be with Yuni, which was my overriding thought that afternoon.

And, with that, I went back to my apartment, although it didn't feel like mine anymore.

I communicated my decision to the people that were listening and prepared a small bag of clothes. The rest of my possessions would be left behind and disposed of by someone.

After checking the room to ensure the gas and air conditioning were working, I received a message (again, I don't know how) that a car would come to collect me at 8 pm. So, with it just being a matter of waiting, I went for a walk and when I got back, it was now dark outside.

Worryingly, many more cars were in the street than usual, so I approached cautiously.

Was it some sort of trap?

Who was I being trapped by?

I felt unsafe and, again, angry for being put in this situation. But I was in this game now and had to be calm and work through my emotions.

The road I lived on ran east-west, and I figured anything to the north would be safe, that being where Ubud was located and where I felt God was watching over me. So I ruled out an attack on me from the north and felt the real danger would be from the south, the direction of Kuta—but there was excellent protection from houses on that side.

I was expecting Yuni to arrive from the west as she would have finished work by now, but that could also be a trap, as she could be used as a pawn to get to me. I hunched down behind a car close to the small shop I knew to be a safe place and waited.

Slowly the cars to the east cleared, so I felt that direction was safe too. But, cars were still parked on the street to the west, which worried me, so I stayed in the shadows and inched closer to my building. I found a place to lie flat on the road under a car that I was certain was empty and watched the road to the west.

Still no sign of Yuni.

I can't recall how I convinced myself I was not under threat, but I eventually did and crept back to my apartment once I was certain the coast was clear. Obviously, there was no danger, but there was a lot at stake now, so I wasn't about to take any chances.

Where was Yuni? I wondered. I walked to Gapet; *maybe she was there with Albert?* To my immense relief, it turned out she was. I was so happy to see her—she was alive and well.

As we talked, I noticed I had developed a new way of talking—very fast and in short sentences. It had come about from when I had been in my room that afternoon when discussing my next mission with my 'bosses', so I needed to revert to normal speech as quickly as possible.

It had been a traumatic day, but now I felt somewhat relaxed and began quizzing Yuni about her previous missions, including that one that had taken her to a dive resort in Sulawesi some years earlier. As best I can remember, I was careful to talk in code as I was still unsure that everything was as I had hoped it to be.

Yuni answered my questions as best she could, no doubt wondering why I was asking about her previous relationship only now, six months into our relationship. And of course, I thought it was obvious—I wanted to know what happened to relationships between secret agents when one person was assigned a new mission.

Once satisfied with her answers, I talked about what I had learned that day before we returned to my room and waited to be picked up. Soon, I saw a car pull up and told Yuni to wait while I checked it out.

And, as I walked down the stairs, I met the person that I least expected to see at that moment—Dad.

Chapter 11: Rage and Endangerment

Even though Dad was the last person I wanted or expected to see that day, his arrival made sense.

It turned out that Yuni had sent an SOS to Rebecca, and Dad was the family member chosen to come to Bali urgently. He had just arrived in France and had to immediately turn around and leave for Bali on two hours' notice. When he arrived, my friend, Dewa, picked him up from the airport and dropped Dad at my place around 8 pm.

I could find his arrival quite logical since he was a secret agent, and now, with what had happened, he needed to be with me to explain everything. I felt an enormous sense of relief, thinking that he would help me understand what the hell was going on.

Even though I didn't show it, I was excited to introduce Dad to Yuni. We sat and chatted outside my apartment for a while, and then Dad suggested it was time for Yuni to go home.

Yuni had more or less been with me non-stop for a week and had done everything in her power to keep me safe. With Dad there to keep watch on me, Yuni went home, leaving Dad and I to walk to Gapet so that he could eat something. We sat down at the table next to the Balinese temple where we would be safe, and I decided there was no point in waiting any longer.

"Who do you work for?" I demanded to know in a tone so aggressive enough that Dad would know it was not a polite enquiry or some kind of dumb joke.

Dad didn't have a clue what I was talking about, but my questions continued.

"You're lying." I said.

He kept a straight face as he deadpanned, "I don't know what you're talking about, Andrew."

I expected Dad to explain how things worked in the world of secret agents and that we would enjoy a brief time together before I left him for my new life. And, when no such explanation followed, I didn't know what to make of it all.

Because Yuni had been communicating with my family, Dad knew I was far from being well, so he might not have been surprised when I said to him I was terrified of losing him. When he questioned me about what I meant, I told him what had happened to me and how I was about to lose him forever.

He had no answers to my questions, and I inevitably stopped asking them.

After we finished dinner, we walked back to my apartment, stopping for ice cream and, by now, I assumed Dad was somehow an innocent victim in all of this. I also assumed that whoever was behind the whole situation would give him the room next to mine—the one previously occupied by Catherine.

But when we returned to my apartment block, there was no sign of anyone, and the other room was locked. Dad was exhausted, and we agreed to go to sleep, sharing my large double bed. The next thing I remember was Dad's phone ringing at around 2 am. He got up, took the call, went to the bathroom, and closed the door.

I was still awake and went to see what was going on, and as I did, I could hear the distinct voice of David. He said something about using a Dutch company, which I assumed was for their yacht purchase, and this sent me into a meltdown.

I became convinced that Dad and David were involved in *The Great Heist*.

Dad finished the call, and despite his protests for me to sleep, I went outside and sat on the balcony. This is the point where the story becomes morbid.

As I sat there, I could see a helicopter in the distance to the south, and I now knew why I had been put through the 'test run' with Yuni a couple of days earlier.

Dad and I were now in serious danger, and it was up to me to see that we averted it. I did not know how safe we were. For example, the apartment to the left was unoccupied but the curtains were closed, so I could not be sure if it was empty.

Perhaps there was a gunman in the room, or maybe it was where Yuni was?

I had no idea.

To the right was the apartment occupied by the Russian lady, and I wasn't sure if she could be trusted. The only thing I knew was that, a few days earlier, I had worked out all the angles, so I knew where the safe spots were in case of gunfire.

As I sat in my seat, with the helicopter off in the distance, a woman walked up the stairs. I desperately hoped it was Yuni, but it was not, and I assumed that women probably had nothing to do with what was going on. With the helicopter still hovering in the distance, I feared for Dad's safety. He was sleeping in the exact position where I knew he could be shot by a sniper in the helicopter.

I told him to move to lie in the other direction of the bed so that his head was out of the way, which he did. I became suspicious when he moved back to his original position.

What is he doing?

All Dad was trying to do was get some sleep, and countless times, he had also asked me to come to bed. But I knew the danger we were now in, so I stayed outside. I was on high alert as I patrolled the space outside my room.

Writing this part is hard because I know what happened; however, putting it into meaningful words is a real challenge.

Essentially, it felt like another test of whether I was up to being a secret agent, not that I needed another one. There were all sorts of emotions going through my mind. As I worked through the game I was now in, I figured that Dad's true colors would become apparent. At some point, he would get up and put a stop to it all.

The game involved yachting terminology, which I was reasonably familiar with. And I believed we were anchored at the center of the world.

I gave Dad a running commentary of how things were progressing outside and gave him many opportunities to intervene and end it. But he didn't move a muscle. And, all the while, I was outside, taking all the risks, and could have been shot at any minute.

Surely, he's going to tell me what to do?

But he never did.

Eventually, I went into my room to boil some hot water, to make a cup of coffee for Dad as I assumed he would be taking over from me on watch, as if we were on a yacht.

But, again, he was unmoved. Outside, the helicopter was gone, and Yuni had not arrived yet.

Was she going to be used as a hostage?

Everything had become so messy, but I still felt calm and in control of the situation. By this time, I had been around the entire building and decided it was secure, other than the room next to mine, from which I still thought I could be shot - the curtains were still draped.

I had been forced into a situation I did not want to be in. Since Dad was not cooperating, I assumed he was willing to die rather than reveal the truth behind *The Great Heist*. I had to decide what to do with him as I now thought of my apartment as a gas chamber—not that it was possible to be one—and not that I wanted Dad to die, either. But, by now, I was beyond angry at the situation.

I locked the door and turned the air conditioning off, and as I did this, Dad sat up and was on his mobile phone. I assumed he was deleting the evidence linking him to *The Great Heist*.

"Stop right there!" I yelled at him, "Or there will be consequences."

Still, at this stage, I felt the situation could be resolved, but that did not happen. I began telling Dad what a bad man he was, that he'd had two failed marriages and had never given a cent to charity. He said we could do something together, but I said it was too late for that.

As I now know, having spoken to Dad about it, he feared for his safety as I talked about putting him in Kerobokan jail and mentioning something about having a gun. And with that, he said he was leaving, and after a short physical struggle on the bed, he walked out the door.

Dad's version is that he escaped, fearing for his safety particularly as the glass doors were flimsy. If our struggle had continued, he feared that we might crash through it.

Mine is that I let him go as I knew he would not get far before the police picked him up and threw him in jail.

So, after Dad left the building, I was on my own once more, and my first thought was - *where is Yuni?*

I figured it was just a matter of waiting—and I waited and waited, but she never arrived.

Chapter 12: Becoming
The Chosen One

Still beyond angry with Dad, I threw his luggage
into the empty lot next to my building and hurled
his expensive watch into the bushes on the other side
of the road.

Fuck him, I thought, wondering why I should reason
with a man who found it plausible to abandon me
when I was searching for answers.

When I felt my surroundings were safe, I glanced
at the clock, and it was nearly 5 am. I set up a table
in view of the CCTV camera outside my door, and
scribbled all the punishments to be handed down
to the culprits behind *The Great Heist* on a piece of
paper . I don't exactly recall the sentences that would
be given, but Dad, David, and Chris were to do time
in the Kerobokan jail. For aiding and abetting them,
Rebecca would, too, serve a week.

I assumed that the entire world could see what
was going on through the tiny lens of a CCTV
camera and, in that moment just before dawn, I

was realizing the significance behind all that was happening around me.

I had saved the world from my evil family, and we would celebrate this victory through a football match between Liverpool and Bali United on July 19th - the day we had previously arranged to celebrate Rebecca's birthday in Bali.

The only people that would be allowed to attend the game would be the Balinese and other Indonesian fans of Liverpool. The match would be broadcast on Indonesian television and radio stations nationwide. Last but not least, it would also be screened in Kerobokan jail for my family and all those involved in *The Great Heist* as a reminder for them of how they had failed.

I laid out chairs on the balcony facing the CCTV camera and thought about who would sit in them. First up, on the good side, was my mate, Tom, who was a Liverpool fan like me. On the other side of the table would be Chris, the evil man, who would be forced to explain his wrongdoings to the world. The next two seats, on either side of the table, were reserved for James and Jamie, my friends who worked under Chris at my old company.

Jamie was red, a Manchester United supporter, while James was white—he was a fan of Tottenham Hotspur. So, I figured I needed to swap them over as both were innocent in *The Great Heist*, although I am still unsure how I reached this conclusion.

I don't know how I reached any of my conclusions during mania. It seems like a complicated thought process, where I provide myself with a logic that reasons with me during the episodes.

The seat at the head of the table was reserved for God, as He would be the ultimate arbiter in the fates of *The Great Heist* culprits. As a figurehead representing God, I reserved that position for Kadek, as a senior village member in Bali. Behind God, on one side would be Mum, and on the other, Yuni.

I realized I needed more chairs, so I went upstairs and took them from outside my neighbors' rooms. With the basics now in place, I began taking things out of my room and placed them on the table, ground, and chairs that I had laid out.

As I write this, I can understand what a comedic script I've laid out in front of you - it wouldn't be a wild idea to suggest that I had lost my marbles. If I could get a recording of that CCTV video, I would look at it day after day and remember just how mad things can get.

Or how hilarious the past can be.

I found a place for more or less every possession I had in my apartment, including all my books. For example, the Dalai Lama's book went on Mum's chair, while *Man's Search for Meaning* went on the chair assigned to Chris. Branson's book went on God's seat as, by now, I reasoned that his connection to Mandela was significant. I also put my Under Armour t-shirt on God's seat to afford him protection.

I think this process took around an hour to complete and, after that, the scene was set.

The next thing I remember was taking the fridge out of my room and putting it on the balcony behind the 'grandstand' of chairs. After all, these VIP guests would need to drink something while watching the match.

The good side was complete, and I began working on the bad side. They would face the other direction, and I symbolized this by hanging my suits, which represented the evil of corporations, on the balcony rail. I didn't need any chairs for the bad side—they could sit on the floor, for that's all they deserved.

The details get a little hazy after this, but I remember setting up my laptop on top of the fridge and pointing it towards the empty lot next to my building, which I had decided would become Jungle Pool.

Jungle was the name of Dad's previous yacht, but I have no idea how it linked to having a swimming pool next door. The whole situation had become completely comical, and I was lapping it up, enjoying my moment in the limelight.

The next part of the story is still vivid in my mind, but it's still hard to shift from my memory to this page. As best as I can remember, I gave a running commentary of the lead-up to the football match while walking on the street outside, and that it somehow involved my nephew, Hugo, who was acting as the producer and roving reporter.

Hugo was innocent in all of this, and he was more capable than adults. I seem to recall talking to Hugo through our headsets while he was reporting on the proceedings from Kerobokan jail—it was total madness.

I then took the water dispenser out of my apartment and placed it in the center of the street. I also hung a broken coat hanger from it as an irrelevant side detail. The world was watching as I stood in the street commentating on the football game. Although the game was due to start, I felt that the world, which had fucked me over, could wait.

I was just wearing a pair of shorts not supporting any side in *The Great Heist*. My Liverpool shirt was on my friend Tom's seat outside my room upstairs. Through cracking the code two days earlier, I had figured out that it all came down to ABC and that it was a formula that could be applied in any situation.

At this moment, A was for Aceh, B was for Bali, but I was not sure what C stood for. Perhaps, it was the Chatham Islands, thousands of miles away to the east? All these things were arbitrary anyway. Aceh was significant as it is known as a place of extreme Islam in the far west of Indonesia, but that didn't bother me. I had no cause for concern for Muslim people - after all, Yuni was one of them.

Eventually, I finished my commentary and told the world it was time for a break. I returned to the balcony outside my room and soon my landlord, Made, arrived around 7 am. I don't know why he came to the building but, no doubt he had been alerted to the fact that there was a problem with a resident. But, as far as I was concerned, nothing was out of the ordinary.

Made was great; we talked, and I expected nothing to come of his visit. But, of course, something came of it—I ended up in the psychiatric ward at Sanglah, a public hospital in Denpasar.

The next thing I remember was there being many people on the street, with me getting tied up by my hands and feet. My head was resting on Dad's blue bag, which had been retrieved from the Jungle Pool, and my red Liverpool shirt was also there.

I felt like a martyr as I was surrounded by Muslims and Hindus as well as men who appeared to be Maoris from New Zealand. I distinctly remember them laughing at me. I was, after all, a freedom fighter sacrificing myself for world peace.

However, in my mind at that moment, the laughter of all these groups of men represented to me that the entire episode had been a joke.

As I lay there, unable to move, I asked for some water and, later, a cigarette, both of which were forthcoming. But, as these things were happening, the men were still laughing at me, or at least that's how it seemed.

From this, I deduced that the whole thing was part of my mission, some kind of setup. There must have been around 30 men on the street at that moment as well as an ambulance.

Eventually, I was untied and began talking about how everyone had underestimated me. On the side of the ambulance were the red and black colors of Canterbury, a sports team from New Zealand that I had supported as a child, so I laughed at the people who thought I was a supporter of New Zealand's 'blue' National Party.

From there, I said that the medical profession was also fraudulent because bipolar was a far too convenient term. I reasoned that we all have ups and downs and anyone could be called bipolar.

But, the most extreme of all, I concluded it was impossible to prove that I was the son of my parents.

So, it was as if I did not even exist and that I could now get on with the thing I wanted more than anything else—to create a life with Yuni and feel free forever.

Chapter 13: Escape from Sanglah

My next memory was being at Sanglah Hospital in Denpasar with Yuni holding my hand and comforting me as I returned to my senses. I don't recall how I got there nor who was with me then, but I was probably drugged and taken by ambulance, possibly even by the police.

Dad had been in contact with Yuni during this time after he spent the early hours of the morning finding a hotel. Yuni and Jero came to my apartment and were told that I had been taken to the hospital. After that, they came to Sanglah to find me.

I distinctly remember looking around the hospital while I was with Yuni and seeing posters on the wall about anti-corruption. I also remember being afraid when the hospital's security staff restrained me.

That was my last memory until I woke up the next morning, strapped to a bed. I had been drugged to put me to sleep, and I was in a room on my own. Well, not quite, as Yuni was also there.

In the middle of the day, she returned to her place to check on her family, before returning to the hospital. Yuni spent that night sleeping on the floor on a yoga mat while I was strapped to the bed. I was so relieved to see her when I opened my eyes in unfamiliar surroundings.

After that, my experience in Sanglah is a total blur. Dad has since told me that the doctors said I wouldn't be able to remember it, which is more or less correct. It was a bit like my time in The Priory in London in 2017, when four weeks seemed to just disappear.

At the point of my psychosis beginning, Yuni and I had been together for six months, and even though Yuni is a single mum with responsibilities for her son and her mum, she kept doing everything she could to ensure I was okay. I can't praise Yuni enough for how she handled the whole situation. She afforded me something that I had not had for seven years—the feeling of love and belonging. Through all of the mania and psychotic thoughts, she was there.

★ ★ ★

I was in Sanglah's psychiatric ward for ten days and it was a vastly different experience from that at The Priory. When I was at The Priory, we were allowed to roam free and mix with the staff; however, at Sanglah, we were kept behind bars.

But, in some ways, I preferred Sanglah.

I felt safer there, much more so than I did at The Priory, where I was genuinely scared of some of the staff. The other patients in Sanglah were Balinese, although one lady from Austria was there, too. This lady had a mobile phone from which I could send emails, connecting me to the outside world.

There were around eight patients at once, and everyone was friendly. Two Balinese girls were nice to talk to, and I kept wondering, in our conversations, what was wrong with them.

The real character of the place was a large Balinese guy who had his own room and was always ordering food from outside, which he shared with us. We called him Big Baby because he was gentle and kind.

After a few days, Sam arrived in Bali to support Dad and Yuni. They worked out a system where Dad and Sam would visit me during the day, and Yuni would come in the evenings after work.

One day, Sam bought me a pair of blue flip-flops, but because of the association with the National Party, I refused to wear them; instead, I kept taking and wearing Big Baby's white pair. This frustrated him immensely, but he never got angry with me.

Yuni's birthday was approaching, and it angered me that I was told that I would not be allowed out to spend it with her as I had planned—a dinner for family and friends at a restaurant in Denpasar. The best I could do was convince one of the staff members to buy Yuni a small cake, which she kindly did.

My recollection of my stay is not very good, but I distinctly remember looking forward to Yuni visiting me each evening. I was less sure about how I felt about Dad, but at some point, my thoughts must have switched to becoming normal again, and the idea of *The Great Heist* disappeared.

It was as if that was never a thing.

As it had been at The Priory, my task now was to escape.

I figured that it would be easy and that it was just a matter of picking the right moment when everyone was asleep, and the staff talked amongst themselves behind the bars separating me from them.

The patient's area was a large compound, and there was a roof that I could easily reach if I balanced two chests of drawers on top of each other. It was just a matter of maneuvering the drawers out of one of the empty rooms and waiting for the right moment to make my move.

I picked Saturday, June 1st, the night of the Champions League final featuring my team, Liverpool. I had pleaded with the staff to let me out to watch the game, but they had refused and I was determined not to miss it.

And so, I climbed out of the compound onto the hospital rooftops and escaped. I knew the area and walked to the Ibis Styles, the same one I'd left my valuables in the week before, where Dad and Sam were staying. I checked in after getting the receptionist to call Sam, who came down to pay for the room.

After going inside my room, I turned the TV on and found the football channel, by which time Liverpool had won the match. I smiled and thought how cool it had been to have beaten the system.

It was probably around 4 am, and after ordering some food, I left my room to scope out the hotel. An Indonesian man was about to leave the hotel and he offered me his cigarettes, the same brand that Yuni smokes. I took this as a positive sign that I was being protected. I walked to the front of the hotel and found two flags, the red and white of Indonesia and another green and white one.

I felt they had been left there for me to find, so I took them to my room and locked them in the safe. What I should have done at that point was go to sleep but, instead, I went back outside. As I lit a cigarette, I noticed many people milling around, and I realized they were the Sanglah hospital staff.

They had found me, my brief vacation was over as I was soon in an ambulance, headed back to Sanglah. I cursed myself for making the schoolboy error of going to the same hotel as Dad and Sam.

Chapter 14: Wild Manic Episode Recovery

I remained in Sanglah until June 7th, when they agreed to release me into the care of Dad and Sam. As I mentioned, the entire experience in Sanglah was a bit of a blur. Mum called the hospital at one point, but I still have no recollection of speaking to her.

Another time I stood in front of the exit door for forty-five minutes so Sam could not leave. He said, "Okay, I guess I'm sleeping here tonight then".

It must have been a bewildering time for Dad and Sam, especially dealing with the hospital staff, who seemed to change daily. However, they did visit Dr. Joy, who told them what to expect—it would take ninety days for me to recover from my extreme mania.

When I left the hospital, I was not fully out of the psychosis, as I seem to remember still suspecting some people on the street in Legian, where Dad had booked rooms for us to stay. But I liked my new surroundings and was happy to be staying close to the beach.

Dad stayed with me for another twelve days, Sam for less, and what's strange about that period is that I don't remember it in the amount of detail as I did when I was in a fully psychotic state. The days just blended into the next as my mind began to calm down.

Dad's primary goal was to get me into a healthy eating routine and return to a normal sleeping pattern. And, of course, getting on a strict regime of taking my medication. When Dad left Bali and headed to France on June 19th to pursue his dream of buying a new yacht, I moved to Ubud, where my Balinese friends were, and I stayed in the upstairs room at my friend Wayan's home.

I stayed there for a week before moving into a small house near Yani's place. It seemed like a good idea to have my own place yet, as I now know, it was a sign that I was still manic at this stage as I soon hated the small house, whereas I liked it at Wayan's place.

Because I was still manic, I was still acting impetuously and began doing things that would immediately compromise my happiness. It wasn't such a big deal, but, for me, it is always nice to be around people, whereas now, I was on my own. Alone with just my thoughts.

Over this period, between coming out of the hospital and the end of June, there's no doubt I was still manic—a quick look back at my emails from that time is proof of that. I sent messages to many people and began impulsively booking random, non-refundable trips to places like China and France that I didn't end up taking.

I also formally ended my employment with English First, and they kindly gave me a good reference. I returned all my teaching materials to the company, even though they had not asked for them—after all, I've always believed in preserving relationships.

The mania wore off in early July when Rebecca and Hugo came to visit but, as happens after a period of mania, I soon became depressed. During this time, my love for Yuni and seeing her a few times a week kept me going.

It is ironic that Dr. Joy had always said that if we could avoid me getting depressed, it was likely that I wouldn't get manic, yet it happened to me the other way round.

In the following months, I moved back to Kerobokan to be close to Yuni, but life felt very different as my new room wasn't as homely as my previous apartment and because I wasn't working.

I was lost with nothing to do each day and, once more, turned to alcohol to get me through this hard time. Inevitably, Yuni told me that I was not taking good care of myself, and she was right. I was a shadow of the man that she loved.

At some point, Yuni and I saw Dr. Joy, and I asked her how I ended up in a state of psychosis.

Her answer was simple, "You pushed yourself too hard, Andy."

After Yuni's stern words, I joined a gym and ate more regularly. I also started teaching English with another company, both in a Bali classroom and online.

It wasn't as enjoyable as at English First, but it gave me a sense of purpose and made me feel alive and well again. Yet, life still felt very fragile.

The one thing that gave me hope more than any other was my relationship with Yuni. By living close to her, we could hopefully go back to how we had been before that fateful moment when I had my first delusional thought.

I hadn't lost my identity, I was still Andrew McLean. Life wasn't perfect but with Yuni by my side, I felt confident that it wouldn't be too long until it felt pretty good again.

"Someone who truly loves you sees what a mess you can be, how moody you can get, and how hard you can be to handle but still want you."

Epilogue

After Rebecca and Hugo returned to New Zealand and before I moved back to Kerobokan to be with Yuni, I spent a few weeks staying in the guest room at Jero's house in Pejeng, a village near Ubud. I wasn't feeling great, but I mustered enough energy to begin making some notes about what had happened to me.

Soon this became a series of emails to friends and family, partly because I had nothing else to do and partly because my manic episode was so bizarre that I thought it might be entertaining for others to read about. I also wanted my family, especially, to know exactly what had happened from my perspective.

What my readers found astounding was the level of detail that I was able to remember two months later, despite my mind being in a state of delusional madness at the time. I did have some help, mainly from Yuni, to clarify certain days and dates or how something happened, but, for the most part, what you've read in this memoir is the action exactly as I remember it.

That was back in 2019, and it's now 2023, and a lot has happened in my life since then. I moved in with Yuni in 2020 but soon became depressed, which led to us breaking up. A lengthy period of depression followed where I was staying in a guesthouse in Ubud with minimal contact with anyone.

Then in September 2020, I went home to New Zealand as Mum's health had deteriorated badly, and I spent six months there. I managed to find a job and stayed with Sam, but it never felt right, so when Mum passed away in February 2021, I moved back to Bali.

On my return, I was determined to find a nice place to live in and in July, I bought a lovely new house in Berawa, which I still live in today. I hadn't had a place to call home for seven years and, boy, what a difference it has made to my mental well-being.

Most significantly, I've been on the same cocktail of medication that Dr. Joy put me on when I initially moved to Bali and guess what? As I type this, it's almost three years without a manic episode. Additionally, it's been more than two years since I have had a prolonged period of depression.

As a New Year's resolution at the start of 2023, being a keen writer, I decided to write my first book, and when I began brainstorming ideas, I realized that I already had the makings of a book with the story I have just told. The only question in my mind was whether anyone would want to hear it.

So, if you have made it this far, and whether you're a medical professional, a sufferer of bipolar disorder, a family member, a friend or just a curious mind, I hope you have found value in my story. And, rather than me rattle off a list of lessons learned, I'll leave you to take from my account what is most pertinent for you.

My main message is that bipolar isn't necessarily a bad thing. Sure, I'd rather not suffer from it, and I wish I could rid myself of it but, regrettably, once we have bipolar, it doesn't go away.

Curiously, what I don't know is how long I have been bipolar for. When I look back at life before The Priory in 2017, there's no doubt that I've had some pretty manic moments, such as when I decided to move to Portugal with no real plan. After two great months there, I returned to London without a job, and all alone - sound familiar?

There's no doubt though, that being bipolar lends itself to having a very creative mind so it's no coincidence that some of the world's most prominent people have been bipolar - actors, musicians, astronauts, film directors, prime ministers and even the founder of CNN.

Just Google 'famous people with bipolar', and you'll be amazed at the list of names. For an excellent documentary, I encourage you to get on YouTube to watch *The Secret Life of a Manic Depressive* by the renowned British actor, Stephen Fry.

I mention Stephen because he talks about a moment where he was right at the point where he could end his life. He had put a hose pipe from his car's exhaust through the window - all he needed to do was turn on the engine but, somehow, he didn't do it.

I've never got that far, but there have been plenty of times when I have thought about wishing I was dead. I think that's a natural reaction for someone like me, whose mood can swing from one pole to the other.

And that's the point of it all - it's about trying to minimize the fluctuations in mood, and the way to do that is by taking medication and having an excellent, trusting relationship with a psychiatrist like Dr. Joy. These days, if I am ever worried about something or need more medication, she is just a What's App message away.

Author's Notes

What is Bipolar Disorder?

You may have noticed that I haven't at any point in this book attempted to define what is bipolar disorder (or 'manic depression' as it is sometimes called) or what behaviors it creates and there's a good reason for that. Simply put, I'm still learning myself and having joined a bipolar support group in Bali recently, it's clear to me that it affects people in different ways, to different degrees.

Instead, I'll try to describe what it can *feel* like when suffering from bipolar disorder, based on what I've felt at times and what other sufferers have told me.

At its peak, a wave of exhaustion hits you, and your mind races with a jumble of thoughts and emotions. You feel overwhelmed, and the day ahead feels like a daunting task. The struggle of dealing with bipolar disorder weighs heavily on you.

With each passing moment, your emotions seem to change, swinging from highs to lows and back again.

It feels like you have no control over the turmoil inside you, and you struggle to keep up with the constant changes. At times, it feels like the darkness will never lift.

But you know that deep down that there is a way out. You yearn for stability and the ability to take charge of your emotions. You want to wake up feeling refreshed and energized, ready to face the day with confidence and positivity.

So if that's you, it's not an easy journey, but you're not alone. With the right support from a medical professional and those people close to you, you can learn to manage your mood swings and take control of your life once again.

Therapy, medication, and healthy habits can all be powerful tools in your arsenal, helping you to create a life that's filled with purpose and joy.

With each step you take, you feel a sense of pride and accomplishment, knowing that you're making progress toward a brighter future. And as you look back on your journey, you realize that the struggles you faced have strengthened you, and made you more resilient, and more determined, than ever before.

So take that first step, reach out for help, and know that there is hope.

The journey may be tough, but the rewards are immeasurable. You have the strength, courage, and resilience to overcome this challenge and create a life that's filled with happiness and stability, with all your loved ones around you, cheering you up.

If you can empathize with what I've gone through, I know how difficult the journey is. I know how terrible it can feel.

It might feel humiliating at some point when you realize that you've made a terrible decision or massively overspent. Or it could also feel like nothing at all, as it does for me much of the time.

The life of a person suffering from bipolar disorder is very, very difficult. But it's not your entire life and you must not let it define you because it's your right to create your own identity.

Life is worth living and many people with bipolar live great lives. And, while I wouldn't say my life is great, it's not too bad either.

So, if I can do it, so can you!

About the Author

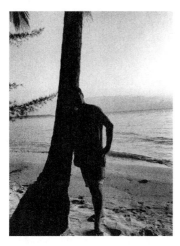

Andrew McLean was born in Wellington, New Zealand, in 1975 and he spent his early years in the Chatham Islands, 300 kilometers to the east of Christchurch, where his dad was a fisherman.

He grew up loving sport and dreamt of being a sports commentator, a dream that was realized at age forty-six, despite the fact he had been diagnosed as suffering from bipolar disorder five years earlier.

He studied law at university in New Zealand and also gained an MBA while living in London, his home of thirteen years and where he was married in 2010. The majority of his career has been spent working in the corporate world, and he's also worked as a journalist and as an English teacher.

He lives in Bali, Indonesia and this is his first book.

Acknowledgments

Creating this book has been a collaborative effort. It started with me writing the initial draft from which Anusha Siddiqui created the manuscript. From there, David Weller edited the book into its final form.

I'm a big believer in the power of collaboration and I'm grateful for the help Anusha and David have given me. I'm certain that this book is a much better read than had I attempted to do it all myself!

Printed in Great Britain
by Amazon

25686475R00086